MOSTLY MACRO

MOSTLY MACRO

A Guide to Healthy Cuisine for the Discriminating Palate

LISA TURNER

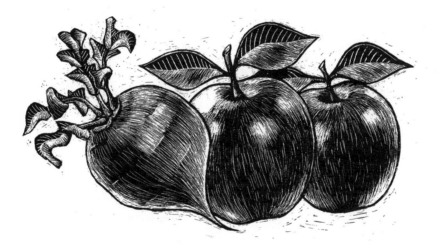

HEALING ARTS PRESS
ROCHESTER, VERMONT

Healing Arts Press
One Park Street
Rochester, Vermont 05767

Note to the reader: This book is intended as an informational guide. The remedies,
approaches, and techniques described herein are meant to supplement, and not to be a
substitute for, professional medical care or treatment. They should not be used to treat
a serious ailment without prior consultation with a qualified health care professional.

LIBRARY OF CONGRESS CATALOGING-IN-PUBLICATION DATA
Turner, Lisa.
Mostly macro : a guide to healthy cuisine for the discriminating palate / Lisa Turner.
p.   cm.
Includes bibliographical references and index.
ISBN 0-89281-534-5
1. Macrobiotic diet. I. Title.
RM235.T86   1995
613.2'6—dc20   94–48512
CIP

Printed and bound in the United States

10 9 8 7 6 5 4 3 2 1

Illustrations by Ian Davis

Text design and layout by Virginia L. Scott

This book was typeset in Sabon with Shelley Allegro Script
and Berling condensed as display typefaces

Healing Arts Press is a division of Inner Traditions International

Distributed to the book trade in Canada by Publishers Group West (PGW),
Toronto, Ontario
Distributed to the health food trade in Canada by Alive Books, Toronto and Vancouver
Distributed to the book trade in the United Kingdom by Deep Books, London
Distributed to the book trade in Australia by Millennium Books, Newtown, N.S.W.
Distributed to the book trade in New Zealand by Tandem Press, Auckland

Accept everything with great pleasure and thanks.
Accept misfortune like happiness, disease like health, poverty like
prosperity, and if you don't like it or cannot stand it, refer to your
universal compass . . . there you will find the best direction.
Everything that happens to you is what you lack.

George Ohsawa

There are no fixtures in nature. The universe is fluid and volatile.
Permanence is but a word of degrees.

Ralph Waldo Emerson

The universe is a friendly place, life is a series of opportunities,
and you can do and be whatever you want.

Felix Bliss

CONTENTS

Part Four

RECIPES

PREFACE

I COME FROM A FAMILY with varying health experiences and diverse interpretations of the notions of nutrition. I come from a family in the South, where fried chicken, vegetables boiled for hours in water and pork fat, and white-flour biscuits constituted a substantial portion of the average daily fare. In the Carolinas, tradition is slow to change, and the unmistakable connection between diet and health receives only tenuous recognition at best, even now.

I mention this as an introduction to and explanation of my own health and some of the factors that led me to write this book. When I was eighteen, I experienced my first bout with what was to be a long and tenacious struggle with kidney problems. I remember waking in the middle of the night, fevered and sweating, with a blinding, burning pain in my abdomen and kidneys. Terrified, I woke my father, who is a physician, and he quickly loaded me up with antibiotics and painkillers. My symptoms were suppressed, and I slept for most of the next forty-eight hours. Three days later, fever down and urine relatively clear, I was permitted to go about my usual routine.

But neither life nor illnesses are so simple. Even as I was lauding the miracles of antibiotics, reveling in my victory over the kidney and bladder battle, my body was quietly rebelling, preparing for an all-out war. Over the next six years I experienced acute attacks of what were diagnosed and then summarily dismissed as bladder infections. During my college years I settled into a dismal health care routine: I plodded off to the student health center every six weeks, entering the doctor's office with urine specimen in hand and leaving with various prescriptions—Keflex, Pyridium, tetracycline,

Tylenol with codeine, Macrodantin—stuffed in my purse; I made monthly visits to the radiology unit for ultrasounds and excruciatingly painful cystoscopies; and as I sat on a hard little chair waiting for the results of my tests, a white-coated doctor leaned across the broad mahogany expanse of his desk and told me that I must undergo surgery to remove endometrial growths or have radioactive dye injected into my kidneys. In spite of the pain, in spite of the time, energy, and money I wasted on countless—and fruitless—doctor's visits and prescriptions, it never occurred to me to question why I was sick.

During all this time, I was following a basic vegetarian diet. I had become a vegetarian at the tender age of twelve, and I was well acquainted with the philosophies of food combining, complementary proteins, and the supposedly necessary inclusion of copious amounts of dairy to compensate for deficient protein—which I included in large quantities indeed. Yet my health continued to decline. I continued to take painkillers and antibiotics and to accept my relentless kidney problems. Everyone has a cross to bear, I figured, and I had found my particular hunk of wood to lug around.

It wasn't until I was twenty-four that I realized I didn't have to hurt all the time. A dear friend, with a long and varied background in natural medicine and nutrition, took me to an Oriental doctor who prescribed herbs, acupuncture, and a radical change in diet. I went through months of herb therapy and acupuncture, and I altered my diet dramatically, completely excluding dairy, chocolate, coffee, caffeine, alcohol, sugar, refined and processed foods, and excess oil and salt. I decreased my intake of liquids and protein as well. It was about that time that I first began reading about and studying macrobiotics. Having nothing to lose at that point, I followed the advice of my Oriental doctor and various macrobiotic practitioners and in time adopted a relatively stringent and rigorous macrobiotic regimen. After following this diet for almost a year, I could count on both hands—with a few fingers left over—the number of kidney flare-ups I'd had.

But life became more complicated, and so did my diet. Whenever I slipped, even in the slightest—a pat of butter, a sliver of Cheddar cheese—my problems returned. I finally realized I was slipping simply because my palate was peeved, bored with the prescribed regimen of brown rice and plain vegetables. At the time, I was cooking professionally and learning a great deal about food and nutrition. I began to experiment, using the skeleton and framework of macrobiotic principles and philosophy, and I created a diet that worked for me. To this day, I follow a diet based on macrobiotic maxims but with some exceptions. And even though I may slip, I rarely actually fall down.

Given all the above, please note that this book is not intended to be a healing regimen based on strict macrobiotic principles. I have a great deal of respect for, and consummate trust in, the traditional macrobiotic diet; I nonetheless believe that for most people, save those few who have serious illnesses or unlimited amounts of time and money, following a strict macro diet is a Herculean—and generally unnecessary—task at best. Thus the premise of this book: Take the best of macrobiotic principles, and adapt them to a Western lifestyle and sense of taste, with fast, simple, and delicious dishes. I won't tell you that macrobiotics will cure you of cancer or chronic fatigue. I do believe, however, that you can create a full, healthy, and more pleasurable life by following a diet that is not completely, but is at least mostly, macro.

Many, many thanks to Adrian Delate and Melanie Melia for their invaluable input and brutal honesty, and to everyone else who read and contributed to this book. All my gratitude to my parents and sister for patiently enduring years of food quirks and quandaries, to my friends for their tasting, testing, and tenacious support, and to Felix Bliss, for being just that.

INTRODUCTION

IN THE EARLY 1960s, George Ohsawa—founder of the macrobiotic movement—introduced macrobiotic principles to the United States. He advocated a diet based on whole grains, vegetables, legumes, and fresh, unprocessed foods, including a small portion of fish, condiments, and other ingredients and excluding sugar and fat. In the ensuing years the macrobiotic diet was too often taken to unnecessary and fanatical extremes, causing skepticism, self-righteous indignation, and outright horror in the orthodox medical community and with the general public, as critics painted a picture of unwashed hippies in tie-dyed T-shirts languishing on futons with bowls of brown rice at their sides.

Now, more than thirty years later, the U.S. government advocates a diet based on whole grains, vegetables and fruits, and small amounts of protein foods, with very small quantities of fats and sugar. These proportions and their philosophy are strikingly similar to the principles espoused by Ohsawa. Americans are now advised to eat high-fiber foods, avoid meat and dairy, limit fat and sugar, and base their diets on grains, beans, and vegetables. The orthodox medical community embraced these recommendations after the U.S. government officially adopted the Food Guide Pyramid in 1992— a move that was based on overwhelming research that pointed out that the foods eaten by the average American caused detrimental health effects.

Even given these findings, macrobiotics is still viewed with some skepticism as an unduly strict and unnecessarily bland regimen based on brown rice and seaweed. Ironically, while the macrobiotic diet is all too frequently perceived as strict and extreme, its focus and intent is, instead, on balance.

In many ways, the currently fashionable fat-free, salt-free diets presented to the American public are far more extreme in their concepts than the macrobiotic diet.

In contrast to the perception of scarcely palatable, pale beige meals of gelatinous white masses of bean curd quivering atop mounds of dry brown rice, the macrobiotic diet includes a stunning variety of colorful beans, grains, vegetables, and condiments that can yield remarkably aesthetic and extraordinarily healthful meals. If you've ever flipped through the pages of a traditional macrobiotic cookbook, you've likely felt the urge to toss the book into a brown-rice pressure cooker and flee to the closest fast-food restaurant. However, a diet that incorporates the most basic, fundamental macrobiotic principles is not only simple and practical, it is also extraordinarily satisfying—and it's a diet anyone can follow, successfully and for a lifetime, with a little tailoring to accommodate personal needs and individual levels of commitment. Herein lies the purpose and plan of this book, which is not about proselytizing or formularizing. You'll find no esoteric mumbo jumbo here—simply a sincere attempt to convey information and inspiration.

The macrobiotic diet was originally conceived as a means of treatment and method of cure for various illness, most notably cancer. After various alterations and modifications, through different schools of practice and thought, a diet has emerged that is intended, for the most part, not as a curative but as a preventive measure, a way of obtaining optimal health.

We are surrounded by a veritable barrage of conflicting information about health, diet, and nutrition, and it has become extraordinarily complicated to make sane choices. And in our hurried and stressful modern lives, what we need most is simplicity and balance. While at first glance the traditional macrobiotic regimen may seem exotic and complicated, a diet based on macrobiotic principles is simplicity itself. In spite of numerous unwieldy texts that carry the principles of the macrobiotic diet to their consummate extremes, thus presenting an unduly rigid regimen, the key principles of macrobiotics embrace the ideal of balance. And in a world where overwhelming stress and a harsh and unstable environment are the norm, balance is the consummate choice—and the only real route to true health.

Please note that many varied, diverse, and sometimes conflicting views on macrobiotics are presented in this book. It is not intended to be a comprehensive analysis of the traditional theories, principles, and practices of macrobiotics—it presents an adequate framework for applying the most essential and vital macro maxims to everyday life.

Excessive theorizing and proselytizing about food is not conducive to creating a harmonious and viable long-term regimen of eating and living.

Dietary habits have as much to do with philosophy and attitude as they do with the pursuit of physical health. Thus if you follow a strict macrobiotic diet but live a life filled with stress, anger, and unhappiness, you can't expect to achieve optimal health on any level—mental, physical, or spiritual. Balance also has to do with the concept that quantity changes quality, or that there is such a thing as too much of a good thing. Also realize that there are many paths up the same mountain, and while your diet and lifestyle may not coincide with the choices made by your friends, family, or colleagues, an attitude of superiority is not in keeping with macrobiotic principles. Balance is rarely achieved through struggle with conflicting ideas and viewpoints.

This book also attempts to convey the idea of respect for food—from appreciating the subtle, imperceptible energy imparted by food to understanding the importance of the tangible, nutritive aspects of food in its quantifiable and measurable nutritional value; from recognizing the importance of respecting the earth and the environment in the production of food to carrying that respect into your kitchen through the way in which food is prepared, presented, and consumed. The idea of respect for food includes the often sadly overlooked reality that food is fuel for the body, a precious reservoir of power and energy that is essential for life. Respect also entails comprehending the concept of waste, including the often superfluous amounts of food prepared and consumed in our modern world and the waste that the consumption of animal products entails in terms of food production and availability on a world scale. On a moral level, macrobiotics acknowledges the concept of respect for the life of the animal itself, in keeping with the macrobiotic principle of a peaceful and balanced existence. Recognize, respect, and have gratitude for the sheer being of food, appreciating it not only as a sensory pleasure but also on a deeper level for the ability it has to maintain and produce life.

And, finally, this book is about personal power and choices, recognizing that you, and only you, have the ultimate ability to decide how you apply dietary principles. Everybody—and every body—is different. No one set of standards and rules can possibly apply to individual physical and psychological makeups. You'll benefit immeasurably when you truly and deeply listen to your body (not the passing and frivolous whims of what your mind tries to tell you your body needs) and trust the advice it gives you—even if it goes against some of the guidelines. When any diet becomes so rigid that it defies your desires and abilities, you'll quickly abandon it from sheer frustration. And when any nutritional practice—macrobiotic or not—becomes exceedingly strict and adheres tenaciously to esoteric philosophies and practices, it will soon be left by the wayside. By relaxing the rules somewhat while still adhering to a diet based on whole, healthy food, you'll be able to follow a mostly macrobiotic diet for life. However you choose to use the theories espoused herein, or in any nutritional practice—macrobiotic or not—recognize that they are your choices, and it's up to you to use them in a way that is most practical, practicable, and pleasurable for your lifestyle. And that's much more than just "mostly" macro.

PART ONE

THE PRINCIPLES OF MACROBIOTICS

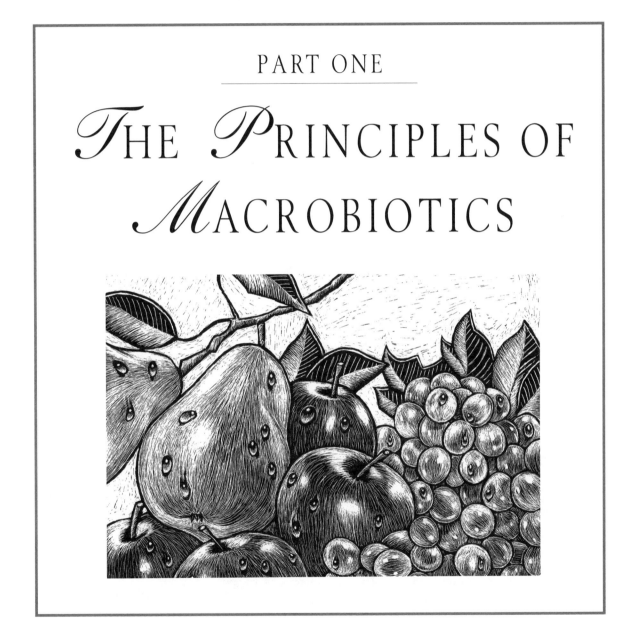

1

HOW OPPOSITES ATTRACT
The Concept of Yin and Yang

WHILE THIS TEXT IS IN NO WAY INTENDED to be a comprehensive analysis of macrobiotic theory, in order to understand the essence of the macrobiotic diet, one must understand the basics of macrobiotic philosophy. The principles of macrobiotic eating and living encompass far more than ingredients, preparation, and presentation. They include aspects of spiritual health and happiness and are a holistic set of beliefs that lay the groundwork for overall health and well-being.

Literally translated from Greek, the word *macrobiotic* means "big life" or "great life"—that is, life as a whole on a larger scale, universal life of the planet, as well as your own life, beyond meals. The Japanese word *Shokuyo* summarizes the principles of macrobiotics quite eloquently: *Shoku* is all matter and energy that creates and nourishes; *yo* is the deed or way to nourish the body. Together the terms translate to mean the right knowledge and actions for creating and sustaining a perfectly healthy body.

The subtle yet fundamental difference between Western and Eastern diets and lifestyles—and, therefore, the perceived difficulties in adopting a macrobiotic-based diet—lie not so much in the shift to unfamiliar foods and preparation techniques as in the diametrically opposed philosophies of West and East. The Western mentality, especially as it pertains to food preparation and consumption, has traditionally focused on the immediate and integral satisfaction of sensory desires. In contrast, the Oriental mentality aims for self-realization of body, mind, and spirit—and food consumption is a central, determining factor in this philosophy. Body, mind, and spirit are fundamentally and constitutionally connected. When you feed your body, you feed your mind and soul.

The Western way is admittedly easier—at least in the short run. It's symptomatic and comfort-oriented, based on immediate gratification and tactile pleasures. After a grueling day at work or a fatiguing fight with a lover, all but the most disciplined of souls are more likely to turn to take-out pizza than a meditation cushion—or a bowl of whole-grain noodles and vegetables that will nourish both body and spirit. This is not meant to imply that you must embrace esoteric religious concepts or undergo immediate spiritual revelations. The point is that a diet—and a lifestyle—based on macrobiotic principles can help restore balance in all aspects of stressful lives.

In Japan eating and drinking are considered a divine art. Compare this to our modern way of thinking and living, composed all too often of fast foods and sensory pleasures. A good meal is one of overabundance; a good restaurant is one from which we often walk away feeling gorged. Western culture has cast aside the importance of simplicity, the concept of balance, and the beauty of careful, thoughtful selection and preparation of ingredients. And in spite of the current trend toward low-fat, low-salt, high-fiber cuisine, our eating habits are still largely based on taste and pleasure, not on healthfulness. In the cacophony of media coverage and cocktail-party conversation about weight loss and quick-fix supplements for various ailments, we've lost our understanding of the importance of and requirements for long-term health; we've lost our appreciation of simplicity and our sense of balance.

YIN AND YANG: THE WAY OF BALANCE

Central to Oriental philosophy is the concept of yin and yang, which is also the governing force of macrobiotics. In macrobiotic philosophy, disease, unhappiness, and all forms of disharmony have one cause: a violation of the order of the universe that causes an imbalance of nature and, consequently, the proper functioning of the body. The essence of yin and yang is somewhat esoteric and difficult to describe in modern terms, but without becoming immoderately simplistic it can be thought of as opposing yet complementary forces that blend and unite to create balance.

The universe strives for harmony, and yin and yang are considered the subtle energetic forces that govern order, working to create symmetry and equilibrium in a world where everything is constantly moving, changing, and shifting. Yin and yang determine the natural order of the universe. Day follows night; spring and summer follow winter; joy follows sorrow. And

THE SEVEN CONDITIONS OF HEALTH
by George Ohsawa

- No fatigue
- Good appetite
- Deep, good sleep
- Good memory
- Good humor
- Clarity in thinking and doing
- Mood of justice; that is, how well you are able to live in harmony with the universe and its constant change.

Though the concept of mood of justice descends from thousands of years of spiritual teachings, it's not so esoteric as it sounds. And you don't have to wear saffron robes or chant mantras in a Zen monastery to attain this lofty goal. The opportunity to practice a "mood of justice" surrounds you in countless, seemingly inconsequential events: The dry cleaner bleaches your silk Chanel suit; the car battery dies five minutes into your trek to the most crucial meeting of your career; the monsoons hit the day of your annual barbecue bash. In macrobiotic practices and Oriental philosophy, these events must be accepted with equanimity and allowed to pass. In other words, take a deep breath, chill out, and relax, because it's not worth the time and effort of fretting about events you can't control.

• Follow a diet based on whole grains, supplemented by a variety of land and sea vegetables, legumes, and small portions of white fish, condiments, and some oils.

• Avoid toxins and poisons from any and all sources—including not only food but also the environment—and consume organic foods as often as possible.

• Eat only what you need, eat only when you're hungry, and stop when you're full.

• Chew food well—at least thirty to fifty times per mouthful—in order to stimulate gastric juices, aid digestion, and help make nutrients in the food more available to the body. Chewing is the first step in digestion and is crucial to assimilation of vital nutrients. As George Ohsawa frequently reminded his students, the intestines don't have teeth.

• Minimize foods from the nightshade family—including tomatoes, eggplants, peppers and potatoes.

• Avoid white sugar and refined flour.

while food, people, and personalities can be characterized as mostly yin or mostly yang, nothing is either one or the other. All entities have a combination of yin and yang characteristics, constantly changing and flowing in an attempt to achieve a state of natural balance.

The concept of yin and yang can best be illustrated by a description of the characteristics of each force. In their most basic incarnations, yin is an expansive, centrifugal force and yang is contractive and centripetal. Yin is related to silence, calm, cold, dark, passivity, responsiveness, inwardness, and decrease, and it is generally thought of as female energy. Yang is related to sound, action, heat, light, movement, activity, excitement, and increase, and it is thought of as male energy. In Oriental philosophy, yin is considered the dark side of the mountain, yang the sunny side of the slope. The concept of yin and yang, while initially somewhat difficult to grasp, is the governing force of the universe and of macrobiotic eating and living. The Japanese have a saying that eloquently sums up the concept of yin and yang: The bigger the front, the bigger the back. The greater the hardship, the greater the happiness that will soon follow. Or, in more Western terms, every cloud has a silver lining, and this too shall pass.

INTANGIBLE ENERGY: YIN AND YANG IN FOODS

The yin and yang concept of balance is the core of the macrobiotic diet. In terms of physical manifestations, yin and yang have many aspects. Every body and personality is made up of a blend of yin and yang characteristics. Some people tend to be more cold-natured or soft-spoken (yin characteristics); others are more warm-blooded and gregarious in temperament (yang characteristics). Softer, rounded bodies are more yin, while lean, wiry builds are more yang. Most people have a combination of both yin and yang characteristics.

The life cycle also encompasses stages of yin and yang: As babies, we possess primarily yang characteristics—we are small, contracted, dense. As we grow and progress into adulthood, yin characteristics become more predominant. We become more expansive, more full and open, taking in and giving off more energy. Then, in old age, yang once again is predominant, as the body begins to contract and becomes harder, smaller, and denser.

The theory of macrobiotics is based on the belief that all foods contain yin and yang characteristics. In the world of modern nutrition, food is thought to be composed of fat, protein, and carbohydrates, as well as vitamins, minerals, trace elements, enzymes, and countless other physically measurable and quantifiable elements. Fats, proteins, and carbohydrates are converted into sources of energy that fuel the body, and vitamins and minerals are cofactors of

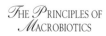

enzymes that control chemical metabolic reactions and allow our bodies to assimilate food for nourishment, building structural components and energy. In macrobiotics, the concept of nutrition in foods is far more complex—and, in many delightful ways, far more simple.

What Makes a Food Yin or Yang?

Everything in nature has a number of specific physical qualities. Likewise, all foods contain specific qualities of yin and yang based on several factors including shape, weight, color, water content, taste, region of origin, and acid/alkaline balance. In general, foods that are yin have a cooling effect on the body, while those that are yang tend to be warming.

Shape
Foods with an expansive, vertical form, or those that grow upward, such as fruits and aboveground vegetables, are generally yin. Those with a lengthened, horizontal form, such as root vegetables, are yang.

Weight
Heavier, denser foods, such as meats, seeds, and most root vegetables, are more yang. Lighter foods like lettuce and leafy green vegetables are yin.

Color
The gradations of color vary and have some exceptions, but in general foods that tend toward the violet, blue, green, and white shades, such as corn and grapes, are more yin. Foods that are in the red, orange, yellow, and brown family, like carrots and pumpkins, are yang.

Water Content
Foods that have a high water content, such as melons, are yin. Those with a low water content, including dry grains, are more yang.

Taste
On a graduated scale, foods that are sweet or sour, like lemons, sugar, and pears, are more yin. Those that have a salty or bitter taste, such as gomashio and some sea vegetables, are more yang.

Regional Factors
Foods from colder climates are yang, while foods from warmer, more tropical climates are yin. Tropical fruits are the most yin and are generally avoided or used in moderation (this concept will be discussed in greater detail later).

- Avoid leavened baked goods and other foods with yeast, which can upset the flora balance in the intestines and digestive system and aggravate candida sensitivities and allergic reactions.
- Drastically reduce your consumption of all sweeteners, dairy, and animal products. According to Ohsawa, sugar and animal protein in excess are the causes of all maladies—both physical and spiritual.
- Avoid alcohol, or use with moderation (about one drink every other day).
- Keep liquid to a minimum (this concept is somewhat controversial and will be discussed further in subsequent chapters).
- Eat regionally grown foods in season as much as possible.
- Make moderate, regular physical activity a part of your daily routine, incorporating the equivalent of about half an hour a day of exercise—anything from a brisk walk to a bicycle ride.
- Keep a healthy, positive mental attitude. Meditate daily, and don't let small worries freak you out.

THE ROLE OF SODIUM/POTASSIUM BALANCE

A less tangible factor in determining whether foods are yin or yang involves the sodium/potassium balance of each food. While this concept is admittedly esoteric, it's also central to the principles of traditional macrobiotics.

George Ohsawa—considered the founder of macrobiotics—was, by most accounts, a sickly child who was afflicted with tuberculosis and other ailments, and he nearly died when he was sixteen. Ohsawa was considered incurable by the doctors he consulted, and when he found he could no longer afford their practices, he refused the recommended cures put forth by his Westernized Japanese family. Instead, he sought the advice and treatment of a doctor in Tokyo named Saigon Ishizuku. According to most accounts, Ohsawa was cured by Ishizuku.

Ishizuku began his studies in the mid to late 1800s, about the time Western medicine was introduced to Japan. He worked as an allopathic doctor in a hospital in Tokyo for some time, but when he became afflicted with a chronic kidney condition, he turned to traditional Oriental medicine and began conducting a series of experiments on himself, introducing various foods into his diet and observing their effects on his health. Over time, and after numerous self-applied trials, he developed a theory based on the importance of the proper balance between sodium and potassium in helping the body assimilate and utilize other nutrients, and he concluded that diet was the chief factor in overall health.

Ohsawa subsequently incorporated Ishizuku's philosophies of cure and his teachings on sodium/potassium balance into his lectures and writings, teaching that food is the cure for illness. In the ensuing years, Ohsawa emphasized the philosophies of living in harmony and incorporating balance into all aspects of life, including diet. He believed that refined white sugar and animal protein in excess are the causes of all maladies—both physical and spiritual—and he suggested that in order to live an ideal life one should eliminate sugar; dramatically decrease animal products; eat primarily grains, vegetables, beans, and seaweed; eat as little as possible of other foods; and keep liquid to a minimum.

Ohsawa arrived in the United States in the early 1960s and started the Ohsawa Foundation in California, which included his clinic, the Sanrant— derived from the combination of the words *sanatorium* and *restaurant* and based on his conviction that all illnesses could be cured by proper diet and lifestyle. After his death in 1966, some of his most notable students, including Michio and Aveline Kushi, continued his work through their macrobiotic centers, writings, and lectures and kept his teachings alive.

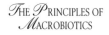

Proportions of Foods in the Macrobiotic Diet

The purpose of introducing the yin/yang theory to food and diet is to promote balance in the daily diet, not to exclude any one category of foods (although there are certain so-called forbidden foods that will be discussed later). Balance is most easily achieved by consuming foods that fall near the center of the yin/yang continuum. It may be argued that the heavy consumption of red meat (which falls in the yang category) and of refined white sugar (which is extremely yin) will conceivably achieve the appropriate balance. In practice, however, this method of achieving balance is obviously neither practical nor advisable. It's like gulping down voluminous quantities of milkshakes or Mexican food for three days straight, then giving up food for the ensuing week: The body, against its will and better judgment, is forced to ricochet continuously between two extremes.

The daily diet can be carefully constructed to ensure a balance of the types, quality, and quantity of foods. This diet needn't entail rigorous preparation and hours of laborious planning, and it doesn't negate the occasional consumption of certain foods in the macro no-nos category. The macrobiotic mandate of balance and proportion involves *attention to* and *awareness of* the daily diet, which is based on grains, vegetables, beans, sea vegetables, unrefined sea salt, unprocessed vegetable oils, and small amounts of seasonings, seeds and nuts, and unrefined sweeteners like barley malt syrup and brown rice syrup.

Dietary needs are never static and fixed; they shift and change constantly, depending on climate, season, health needs, body composition, age and gender, and activity level. Even daily weather fluctuations affect the body's need for certain foods. Though it may be painfully obvious, you'll probably want and need more protein foods, hot dishes, and hearty stews if you're cross-country skiing in the Alps in January than if you're prowling the streets of New Orleans in the middle of July.

In the traditional macrobiotic diet, grains compose 50–60 percent of the daily diet, vegetables about 25–30 percent, beans and bean products about 10 percent, sea vegetables about 5 percent, and soups about 3–5 percent. Animal foods, such as fresh fish, are eaten two or three times a week. Seeds, nuts, and spreads or butters made from seeds or nuts are consumed in small amounts (one to two tablespoons a day) as snacks or condiments. Fresh, unprocessed, locally grown fruit is eaten a few times a week, and tropical fruit is strongly discouraged, except in very warm climates or in the hottest of summer months. Naturally processed and unrefined oils are used in small amounts for cooking or seasoning—the generally recommended quantity is one to two tablespoons a day.

Condiments—including gomashio, seaweed powder, umeboshi, and tekka (these terms will be explained soon)—are used in small amounts to provide seasoning and balance to meals. Pickles made from daikon, turnips, cabbage, or other vegetables are included in small amounts to stimulate the appetite and aid in digestion. Beverages such as spring or well water, bancha tea, roasted grain teas and coffees, and other nonaromatic root or herbal teas are also consumed in small amounts—about two to four cups a day. Again, these proportions often fluctuate, given seasonal and personal changes and needs.

The heavy emphasis on grains in the macrobiotic diet—about half of the daily diet—closely parallels the recommendations set forth by the U.S. government and most knowledgeable nutritionists. Throughout most of history, the human diet has consisted of a diet of legumes, vegetables, and, most notably, whole grains—foods that are rich in protein, complex carbohydrates, vitamins, and minerals. The roller mill was invented around the turn of the twentieth century, and thus began the demise of the humble and virtuous grain. Commercial interests and profit motives prevailed, and denuded wheat in the form of finely textured white flour became all the rage. The roller mill allowed the exterior bran and germ portions of whole grains to be separated from the endosperm, primarily for aesthetic purposes and to help keep the grains from going rancid without refrigeration. Essential oils, trace minerals, enzymes, and fiber exist in the bran and germ, and the refining process removes these crucial nutritional elements. Consequently, the macrobiotic diet uses only whole grains, which contain the ideal proportions of complex carbohydrates, fats, proteins, vitamins, and minerals.

Whole grains provide abundant fiber, which has been recognized as a factor in reducing the risk of many types of cancer. British researcher Denis Burkitt found in the early 1970s that the rates of heart disease, obesity, and gastrointestinal disturbances were lower in Asia and Africa—countries with a higher consumption of fiber—than in Western countries. Other research involving cultures that consume high quantities of complex carbohydrates and whole grains indicates that whole grain–based diets are related to a lower risk of heart disease. Countless studies have shown that the consumption of complex carbohydrates and whole grains can aid in weight control. Whole grains are nutritionally superior to the bland, pale, highly refined flours that have become ubiquitous in American food preparation—they're rich in B vitamins, vitamin E, phosphorus, and other minerals. And they're relatively cheap and eminently versatile.

Disparate interpretations and opinions exist regarding the proportions of various types of foods in the traditional macrobiotic diet. The most generally accepted proportions in the strict macrobiotic diet are those set forth by Ohsawa in what he called his "10 Regimens to Health and Happiness," an admittedly rigorous plan that addresses the proper proportions of various foods (Table 1). According to Ohsawa, the ideal level of physical, mental, and spiritual health is achieved at Level 7, though most of us in the modern world hover around Level 1 or sink into the theoretically disreputable negative notches. Try for Levels 4 through 6 if you're wildly optimistic about your degree of self-discipline and ability to resist various and sundry temptations. More realistically, if you base your daily diet around the proportions recommended at Level 3, dipping into Level 2 every once in a while with the occasional inclusion of animal products (such as fish), salads, and fruit, you'll likely fare better.

Table 1
10 REGIMENS TO HEALTH AND HAPPINESS

LEVEL (%)	CEREALS* (%)	VEGETABLE (%)	SOUP (%)	ANIMAL (%)	SALAD/FRUIT (%)	DESSERT (%)
7	100					
6	90	10				
5	80	20				
4	70	20	10			
3	60	30	10			
2	50	30	10	10		
1	40	30	10	20		
–1	30	30	10	20	10	
–2	20	30	10	25	10	5
–3	10	30	10	30	15	5

* Percentages reflect relative proportions of food in the daily diet.

Obviously, Ohsawa's recommendations needn't be followed so literally. They merely indicate what the founders of macrobiotics considered the "perfect" diet. Rigorous adherence to this intimidatingly strict formula is neither practical nor advisable. It's possible to create a middle ground, a diet that applies the best of traditional macrobiotic maxims and wisdom to modern needs and desires. In the simplest of terms, if you make grains the center of your meal, with vegetables and small amounts of protein foods, simple soups as appetizers, and small quantities of condiments (such as nuts, seeds, miso, gomashio, and pickled vegetables), you will successfully straddled the line between macrobiotic ideals and modern practicality.

AVOIDING EXTREMES:
THE MIDDLE ROAD

In Oriental theory, a good appetite is a sign of overall health, and it indicates happiness, contentment, and peace. Unabashed gluttony is obviously not encouraged by the macrobiotic principle. Food is fuel for the body, and macrobiotic practices encourage curbing the appetite and eating slowly and thoughtfully just until full. Chewing each mouthful at least thirty times, ideally until the food is liquefied, helps to mechanically break down the food, making it easier to digest. It also stimulates the secretion of gastric juices. And thorough chewing causes the jaw to tire, naturally decreasing and discouraging excessive food intake. In general, disease is seen as a sign of excess, and rarely a deficiency, in eating habits. The macrobiotic philosophy is based on the concept of eating and drinking the necessary minimum, remembering that quantity changes quality and that individual needs are different.

Ideally, the diet should consist primarily of foods that tend toward the center of the yin/yang scale, and each meal should incorporate both yin and yang foods for the consummate macrobiotic balance (Table 2). In practice, this creates a diet that is both flexible and extraordinarily easy to follow. The recipes and meal plans in this book are based on balancing yin and yang foods in each meal. As you become more familiar with foods that are yin and yang in nature, you can be creative in designing your own meal plans that are balanced, flexible, and satisfying. As Wendy Esko writes in *Introducing Macrobiotic Cooking*, "The sooner you learn common sense and intuition, the better and more efficient your cooking will become. Once you know the proportions, begin experimenting with different combinations of food. Be creative and artistic. . . . Trust your senses instead of utensils."

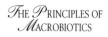

Table 2

EXTREME YIN AND YANG FOODS
AND MODERATE FOODS

EXTREME YIN FOODS

Tropical fruits/nuts: bananas, brazil nuts, cashews, coconuts, figs, grapefruit, hazelnuts, kiwi, lemons, mangoes, oranges, papayas, pistachios, tangerines

Dairy foods: butter, cheese, cream, ice cream, mayonnaise, milk, yogurt

Other sweeteners: corn syrup, honey, molasses, saccharine, sugar

Alcohol

Spices

EXTREME YANG FOODS

Eggs

Meat and poultry

Red-meat fish and seafood: salmon, swordfish, tuna

MODERATE FOODS

White-meat fish and seafood: carp, clams, cod, flounder, haddock, halibut, oysters, red snapper, scallops, shrimp, sole, trout

Whole grains: barley, brown rice, buckwheat, corn, couscous, millet, oats, rye, sweet rice, wheat

Nuts and seeds: almonds, filberts, peanuts, pecans, poppyseeds, pumpkin seeds, sunflower seeds, walnuts

Beans and bean products: azuki (aduki) beans, black beans, garbanzo beans (chickpeas), kidney beans, lentils, lima beans, navy beans, pinto beans, soybeans, split peas, tempeh, tofu, seitan, soy cheese

Sea vegetables: arame, dulse, hijiki, Irish moss, kombu, nori, wakame

Root/stem vegetables: burdock, carrots, cauliflower, daikon, onion, parsnips, pumpkin, radishes, rutabaga, green beans, summer squash, turnips, winter squash

Green vegetables: broccoli, Brussels sprouts, cabbage, celery, Chinese cabbage, chives, collard greens, cucumber, endive, kale, leeks, lettuce, mustard greens, parsley, peas, scallions, Swiss chard, turnip greens, watercress

Temperate fruits, fresh and dried: apples, apricots, blueberries, cantaloupe, cherries, grapes, peaches, pears, plums, raisins, raspberries, strawberries, watermelons

Grain/fruit sweeteners: barley malt syrup, fruit juice, brown rice syrup

2

MODERN LIFE AND THE MACROBIOTIC MANDATES

SINCE THE TURN OF THE CENTURY, most of the foodstuffs in the American diet have undergone tragic changes and adulterations. Food processors began refining whole grains for commercial and aesthetic purposes, removing the nutritionally valuable outer portions of whole grains. Produce is heavily treated with preservatives to allow it to be transported across the country. The soil has been drastically depleted of vital nutrients through modern, chemical agricultural techniques, resulting in significant decreases in the nutritional value of foods. A 1994 study by Doctor's Data, a research laboratory based in Chicago, examined the differences in nutritional content between organic and commercially grown foods, comparing the levels of twenty-six minerals in five foods. The study found that mineral levels are dramatically higher in organic foods—for example, the average levels of calcium and manganese were more than 400 percent higher in organic than in commercially grown foods.

Sadly enough, the use of chemical pesticides and fertilizers to increase crop yield and size has increased dramatically. According to the 1993 National Coalition Against the Misuse of Pesticides report, it was estimated that more than 800 million pounds of pesticides were used to grow food in the United States, and agricultural pesticide use has increased 170 percent since 1976. According to Environmental Protection Agency (EPA) estimates, pesticide residues on food could account for about 6,000 cases of cancer every year. In its 1989 report entitled *Alternative Agriculture*, the National Research Council noted that commonly used insecticides, herbicides, and fungicides have been found to cause tumors in laboratory animals. Currently, about three hundred pesticides have been approved by the federal government for use on food crops. Out of those three hundred pesticides, seventy-three are considered probable or possible carcinogens. In short, what we have been left with is food that is substantially nutritionally inferior to what our ancestors ate a century ago.

In terms of the dietary habits of Americans, meat and animal protein intake has increased while the quality of animal foods continues to decline as a result of the use of hormones, antibiotics, preservatives, and other chemicals. The consumption of processed foods, artificial ingredients, chemicals, additives, and refined sweeteners has increased, as has the intake of fats, especially saturated fats from animal products. Meanwhile, the consumption of fiber has generally decreased.

MODERN DISEASES AND IMBALANCES RELATED TO DIET

It's no wonder that while the average life span has increased in the United States, overall health is dismally low and continues to decline at an alarming rate. The World Health Organization (WHO) in 1992 ranked the United States eighteenth in the level of "good health" among developed countries. In 1990 the United States ranked ninth in mortality rates for men and eleventh for women—a decidedly dubious standing, given that the United States is considered by some to be the most advanced nation on the planet. Japan ranked first in 1993 among countries whose citizens were born with the longest life expectancy, with an average of almost seventy-nine years. According to the 1994 "Prevention Index," *Prevention Magazine*'s annual survey of 1,250 adults, the overall health score for Americans that year was about 67 out of a possible 100.

The cost of the continuous and often fruitless search for health through modern medicine is exorbitant. Economists predict that national health care expenditures as a share of gross domestic product for the United States will rise from 14 percent in 1992 to 18 percent by the year 2000, possibly soaring to 32 percent by the year 2030. The United States spends more of its gross national product on health care than any other country. Americans spend thousands of dollars per year on the cure and treatment of common ailments such as cancer, allergies, diabetes, heart and circulatory diseases, and mental illness. About 70 percent of the U.S. health care budget is spent on the symptomatic treatment of chronic degenerative disease, without addressing underlying causes. These figures become all the more tragic in light of the 1988 Surgeon General's Report on Nutrition and Health, which identifies diet as the single most significant factor in preventing heart disease and cancer.

Cancer

The second leading cause of death in the United States is cancer, killing more than half a million Americans yearly, despite the lavish sums of money and exorbitant human resources spent on research for cancer cures. Since the federal government announced its official war on cancer in 1971, approximately $1 trillion have been spent on researching and attempting to cure cancer, all to no avail. So great has been the failure that in the mid 1980s the *New England Journal of Medicine* called the war on cancer a "qualified failure."

According to the January–March 1994 *Statistical Bulletin* from the Metropolitan Life Insurance Company, the decrease in mortality rates from all forms of cancer has been relatively small over the past few decades, and overall cancer rates in the United States have slowly increased. Deaths from cancer have risen more rapidly than total deaths in the United States, according to the *Statistical Bulletin:* At the turn of the century, the cancer rate was about 1 in 25; in 1994 it was about 1 in 4. Between 1950 and 1990, U.S. death rates from respiratory cancer rose dramatically among women, increasing almost sixfold, while respiratory cancer rates among men nearly tripled. In comparison, cancer mortality rates among Japanese women declined by almost 14 percent.

Gladys Block, an epidemiologist at the University of California, Berkeley, reviewed more than 150 vitamin studies and found that the rate of many cancers is almost twice as high among people who do not regularly consume fruits and vegetables. In addition, researchers from the National Cancer Institute studied 30,000 people in the Henan Province in China—an area that has the highest rates in the world of certain types of cancer—and found that the study group that received a combination of vitamin E, beta carotene, and selenium showed a lower rate of death from cancer.

Additional compelling information regarding phytochemicals has come under recent scrutiny. Phytochemicals are compounds found in food and are believed to help protect against cancer. Garlic, onions, and leeks contain allium compounds, which may decrease the reproduction of tumor cells. Members of the cruciferous family (broccoli, bok choy, Brussels sprouts, cabbage, cauliflower, turnips, and certain greens) contain indoles, which may reduce the risk of breast cancer. Soy products and dried legumes contain protease inhibitors, which may slow the growth of tumors; phytosterols, which may prevent colon cancer; isoflavones, which may reduce the risk of breast or ovarian cancer; and saponins, which may prevent cancer cells from multiplying. Sadly enough, it was estimated that in the late 1980s, the average American consumed less than one cup of vegetables a day and less than half a cup of legumes.

Cardiovascular Disease

Cardiovascular disease, including heart attacks, strokes, and circulatory disorders, remains the leading cause of death in the United States. In 1992 an estimated 722,000 people died from cardiovascular diseases, accounting for one-third of all deaths, and about 300,000 coronary bypass operations were performed at a cost of about $40,000 each. About 50 million Americans have high blood pressure.

Americans experience substantially higher death rates from cardiovascular disease than their counterparts in other countries. According to 1990 figures, Japanese males had the lowest death rate from cardiovascular disease; men in France, Switzerland, Canada, and Iceland had death rates at least 25 percent lower than men in the United States. The statistics for women are similar: In general, the death rates from heart disease for women in other countries remain much lower than for women in the United States.

Fat and cholesterol have been implicated in many types of cardiovascular disease. The highly publicized Framingham Heart Study, begun in the mid 1950s, found that over the course of thirty-five years none of the subjects in the study with a cholesterol level lower than 150 mg had a heart attack. The national average cholesterol level in 1993 was 211 mg.

United States Department of Agriculture (USDA) recommendations call for a diet that consists of a fat intake of 30 percent or less of total calories; some nutritionists recommend reducing fat intake to 15–20 percent of total calories. Most nutritionists estimate that daily fat intake in 1994 constituted 37 percent of the average American's diet. Findings from the China Diet and Health Project—a collaborative effort among Cornell University, the Chinese Academy of Preventive Medicine, and Oxford University, begun in 1983 to evaluate the relationship between diet, lifestyle, and disease—indicate that a diet based on plant foods, with levels of no more than 10–15 percent of total calories from fat, is most likely to reduce the chances of cardiovascular disease and various cancers.

To calculate the maximum amount of fat you should consume on a daily basis, multiply your total daily caloric intake by .15 (or by .10) to yield the total number of fat calories generally in keeping with a mostly macro diet. To determine the grams of fat, divide that number by 9—the number of calories per gram of fat.

Obesity

Obesity—defined as weighing more than 10–20 percent above one's ideal weight—is categorized as the leading health problem in the United States. According to the "Prevention Index," diet and weight control were the biggest health challenges for the nation in 1994, as Americans began to tire of low-fat, sugar-free diets. About 68 percent of adults twenty-five years of age or older exceeded the recommended weight, according to the Index, and

CALCULATING FAT INTAKE

```
  1,800   (total calories/day)
×   .15   (percent of daily diet
          consisting of fat calories)
  ─────
    270   (fat calories per day)


    270   (fat calories per day)
÷     9   (calories per gram of fat)
  ─────
     30   (grams of fat per day)
```

only one in five fell within the recommended range. More than 65 percent of the adult population in the United States begins a new diet every year. One 1989 survey by the *American Journal of Public Health* found that 40 percent of almost 15,000 women nationwide, and 25 percent of almost 7,000 men, said they were currently trying to lose weight and that they were trying to lose an average of thirty pounds.

Other Diseases

According to *Macrobiotic Diet* by Michio and Aveline Kushi, 73 percent of Americans suffer from headaches and 50 percent suffer from such common ailments as backaches and muscle and joint pain. Almost 13 million Americans have birth defects; some infectious diseases—including tuberculosis and syphilis—have reached epidemic proportions, and new strains of bacteria and viruses continue to develop; and about 29 million Americans—nearly 1 in 5 adults—suffer from serious mental illness.

DAILY DIET CULPRITS AND THE BASIC MACROBIOTIC DIET

There's no mystery about the origin of our health woes. Numerous studies have addressed a number of dietary culprits that directly influence health, in both the long term and the short term: high-fat diets, excess sugar, low fiber intake, and excessive consumption of animal products are the primary culprits. The principles espoused in the basic macrobiotic diet are exquisitely suited to avoid many of these maladies by naturally reducing the consumption of so-called dietary demons.

Fats and Oils

Despite heavy media coverage and numerous, ominous warnings from the medical community regarding the detrimental effects of excess fats, the average American continues to consume a diet that consists of about 37 percent fat. In contrast, the USDA recommends that calories from fat constitute no more than 30 percent of the diet, and some nutritionists advocate a consumption of closer to 10–20 percent.

In the macrobiotic diet, fats and oils are used sparingly: About one to two tablespoons per day are used for cooking, a small quantity of nuts and seeds are allowed, and the negligible amounts of fat inherent in grains and legumes are considered. A conservative estimate places total fat calories between 200 and 400 calories per day. Assuming a diet of 1,800–2,400 calories per day, this amount falls well within the USDA's 30 percent guideline, leaning more toward the 10–15 percent recommendation.

In practical terms, radically reducing fat intake is quite simple on a macrobiotic diet. Most recipes use about two teaspoons of oil for cooking purposes. If you concoct three recipes per day, taking into account the small amounts of fat in beans and grains and the moderate use of nuts and seeds, the transition to a low-fat diet can be virtually painless (Table 3).

As your diet changes to one based on grains, vegetables, legumes, and other whole foods, you'll be drastically reducing—or ideally eliminating—the use of processed foods on a daily basis. When you cut cheese fries and chocolate-chip-cookie-dough ice cream from your regular regimen, daily fat intake will be automatically and significantly reduced. And you'll further lower your fat intake by eliminating dairy and meat. (Remember that the diet advocated by this book is not fat free, nor does it forbid indulging in the occasional canapé at cocktail parties or special dinners. Intermittent indulgence is allowed here—and even encouraged. The focus is on balance.)

Table 3
CALORIE AND FAT CONTENT OF FOODS

FOOD SERVING	CALORIES	FAT (GRAMS)
Chicken (4 ounces)	253	13.6
Tofu (4 ounces)	160	8
Tempeh (4 ounces)	224	8.8
Cheddar cheese (1 ounce)	110	9
Soy cheese (1 ounce)	70	5
Cream cheese (1/2 cup)	434	44
Sour cream (1/2 cup)	208	20
Butter (1 tablespoon)	102	3.8
Margarine (1 tablespoon)	102	3.8
Vegetable oil (1 tablespoon)	120	4.5
Peanut butter (1 tablespoon)	100	8
Tahini (1 tablespoon)	90	8
Mayonnaise (1 tablespoon)	110	12
Tofu mayonnaise (1 tablespoon)	40	4
Whole-grain noodles (1 cup cooked)	174	0.6
Black beans (1 cup cooked)	226	1
Brown rice (1 cup cooked)	218	1.6
Almonds (1 ounce)	167	14.8

The types and sources of fats and oils used in the diet are crucial. High-quality fats and oils are nutritionally necessary. Stored fat provides an accessible source of energy, surrounds and protects organs, and acts as an insulator to keep the body warm, and the body uses fatty acids to store energy. In addition, polyunsaturated fats contain fatty acids that are essential for synthesizing hormones, making fat-soluble vitamins (such as vitamins A and D) available to the body, and maintaining cell membranes. Essential fatty acids (EFAs) play a crucial role in preventing cardiovascular disease by virtue of their role in the transportation and metabolism of cholesterol and fats in the blood. The two EFAs are linoleic acid and alpha-linolenic acid. Linoleic acid is fairly common and is found in oils, nuts, seeds, whole grains, and legumes, while alpha-linolenic acid is less common, since it is easily destroyed by processing. Alpha-linolenic acid is associated with decreased risk of tumor formation and heart disease.

Fats and oils vary in terms of nutritional value. Saturated fats, which are solid at room temperature and are found in red meat, cheese, butter, palm kernel oil, and coconut oil, have been implicated in the development of cardiovascular disease and some cancers. A 1994 study by a Yale University researcher at the University of Toronto found that eating 10 grams of saturated fat a day may raise a woman's risk of ovarian cancer by 20 percent. By way of comparison, the average American eats about 30 grams of saturated fat a day, mainly from animal products and processed foods.

The best sources of fatty acids are those obtained from monounsaturated or polyunsaturated oils such as unrefined sesame seed, sunflower, safflower, corn, and olive oils (Table 4). All oils should be unrefined, minimally filtered, and pressed at low temperatures. Read labels for this information, and beware of the term "cold-pressed"—it's often a marketing ploy, since only olive oil and a few other oils can be extracted without the use of heat.

Hydrogenated oils should also be avoided, since the process of hydrogenation—used to make polyunsaturated oils solid at room temperature, as with margarine—converts polyunsaturated oils to saturated fat. The hydrogenation process creates what are known as trans-fatty acids, which have been shown to increase low-density lipoprotein (LDL) cholesterol levels to the same degree that saturated fat does. LDLs contribute to hardening of the arteries and platelet aggregation. High-density lipoproteins (HDLs), on the other hand, help keep blood fats at healthy levels. The Harvard Schools of Public Health announced in 1993 that margarine can increase the risk for heart disease by as much as 70 percent in women. An article in the *American Journal of Public Health* in 1994, written by Harvard nutritionist Walter Willett, reported that margarine and other processed foods could be the cause of 30,000 of the country's approximately 750,000 yearly deaths from cardiovascular disease.

Table 4
AMOUNTS OF MONOUNSATURATED, POLYUNSATURATED, AND SATURATED FATS IN OILS

OIL	% FAT		
	Monounsaturated	Polyunsaturated	Saturated
Almond	65	26	9
Butter fat	30	4	60
Canola	60	34	6
Corn	27	60	13
Olive	82	8	10
Peanut	51	30	19
Safflower	13	79	8
Sesame	46	41	13
Soybean	28	58	14
Sunflower	19	69	12

Sugar

The history of sugar is a long and convoluted one. The refined white substance we know as sugar today first became popular more than 1,300 years ago. Arabs began the widespread trading and commerce of refined sugar when they embarked on long expeditions with sugar for trade. They introduced much of the developed world to the then-unfamiliar taste and mild stimulating effect of refined sugar.

Under the papacy, Europeans began growing, refining, and trading sugar, recognizing considerable profits and gustatory pleasures. They soon realized that to sell sugar, they had to have access to, and control over, regions in which sugarcane was produced—that is, regions with warmer climates, especially on the African continent. It is said that the Crusades were initiated in part for control of the ever-growing sugar trade, as Europeans realized the profitability in gaining control of regions in which sugarcane was produced.

When Christopher Columbus began his journey to America, he loaded up his ships with sugar, which was by then in great demand. Several centuries later, when slaves were brought to America, one of their primary assignations was to grow and harvest sugarcane. Thus began America's considerable, if somewhat tragic and excessive, love affair with refined white sugar—in 1993 the average American consumed more than 130 pounds of sugar per year.

Much controversy has surrounded this all-pervasive substance over the past two decades. The battle lines have been decisively drawn between those who rigorously maintain that sugar is a relatively innocuous substance and those who proclaim it "white death," linking it to tooth decay, hyperactivity, high blood pressure, diabetes, obesity, and mental disorders. The body's speedy uptake of refined white sugar disrupts the normal release of insulin levels and affects the liver's glucose response, stressing the pancreas and adrenals. And some research has linked excessive consumption of sugar to manic behavior, schizophrenia, and depression. A 1993 study at Texas A&M University found that when a test group of subjects who suffered from major depression were placed on a diet that banished refined sugar, the group's scores on standard depression tests were significantly improved after only three weeks.

Some nutritionists maintain that refined white sugar is the same as honey, brown rice syrup, molasses, and other sweeteners. Since all are chemically converted into glucose during the metabolic process, they say, the body is unable to recognize the difference. While this point has a certain scientific validity, it does not take into account a number of other factors. Refined white sugar, from which vital minerals, nutrients, and trace elements are removed during the refining process, depletes nutrients in the body, especially chromium, zinc, calcium, vitamin C, and vitamin B. It reduces digestive enzymes and hydrochloric acid, a digestive aid in the stomach, thus disrupting the digestive process. Refined white sugar is metabolized quickly, causing sharp fluctuations in blood sugar levels, which can lead to hyperactivity, depression, and other mental disturbances.

The macrobiotic diet eschews white sugar entirely and substitutes high-quality natural sweeteners, especially grain-based sweeteners such as barley malt syrup, brown rice syrup, and amasake. Mirin, maple syrup, and honey are used on occasion, and sweeteners of tropical origin, such as molasses, date sugar, and sugarcane, are generally avoided as are artificial sweeteners, for obvious and well-publicized reasons. All sweeteners are used in moderation, primarily because sweeteners—whether brown rice syrup or refined white sugar—are considered extremely yin, and most disease and dietary woes are said to arise from an excess of yin. According to macrobiotic philosophy, some of the most likely causes of yin disease are refined foods, soft drinks, wine, beer and alcohol—all products with a high sugar content. If you're in overall good health, an after-dinner mint or occasional cookie won't hurt you, but you're better off using grain sweeteners on a regular basis—and you'll be surprised at how rich and flavorful brown rice syrup and barley malt syrup taste compared with refined white sugar.

Fiber

The U.S. government adopted the Food Guide Pyramid in 1992, the new set of dietary guidelines that replaced the traditional Four Food Groups as the mainstream standard and recommending that 50 percent of the daily diet be composed of whole grains and grain products. Yet most Americans have not substantially changed their eating habits. Surveys indicate that the average American still consumes only about three servings of grains per day, compared with the six to eleven servings recommended by the Food Guide Pyramid.

Numerous studies have reinforced the nutritional significance of a high-fiber diet, while low-fiber diets have been implicated in everything from heart disease to cancer to obesity. Dietary plant fiber has been shown to help lower blood cholesterol levels and protect against cancer—most notably, colon and breast cancer—as well as gallbladder disease, ulcers, and other digestive disorders. In 1991 a study commissioned by WHO, entitled *Diet, Nutrition and the Prevention of Chronic Diseases,* noted that the modern diet contains only one-third of the fiber intake of preceding generations. The study set optimal total dietary fiber intake at 40 grams per day.

Fiber is crucial for effective digestion and assimilation of nutrients and for elimination of waste products. Plant cells are surrounded by a wall of complex carbohydrates—including lectins, pectins, and starches—which are not assimilated by the body. Unlike fats, proteins, and simple carbohydrates, which are absorbed almost entirely in the small intestine, fiber is not digested and moves through the large intestine virtually unaltered, adding bulk to fecal matter and facilitating its rapid transit through the colon, thus inhibiting the formation of toxins and bacterial growth. There are two types of fiber in plant materials—insoluble and soluble. Insoluble fibers help soften fecal matter, thus speeding elimination. Soluble fibers include gums found in beans, oats, corn, and barley; mucilage found in seeds; and pectins found in fruits. Soluble fibers reduce cholesterol levels and blood lipids, help stabilize blood sugar, and speed the excretion of bile acid.

In the mid 1980s, when oat bran was found to help decrease blood cholesterol levels, the fiber craze, fueled by widespread media attention, caught on like no other cultural food fondness since sushi. After several months, oat bran began to wane in popularity as Americans realized that they could eat only so many bowls of bland and gritty gruel for breakfast. Rice bran quickly followed on the heels of oat bran; it also made a rapid descent, for many of the same reasons. After trying to incorporate bran into everything from muffins to soup stocks, the average American gave up and went back to bagels for breakfast.

The macrobiotic plan, based on a diet composed of 50 percent whole grains and 25–30 percent vegetables, is naturally high in fiber. Elaborate and cumbersome meal planning to incorporate the recommended 40 grams of fiber into the daily diet isn't necessary. In a balanced macrobiotic diet, it's already there.

THE MEAT MYTH

It's a common misconception that vegetarians are sadly deficient in protein. Concern and eyebrows have been raised among old-school nutritionists regarding the lack of protein and B vitamins in a vegetarian—especially vegan (dairy-free)—diet. After all, most of us were raised with the Four Food Groups mentality, and ever since grade school, we've listened to various forms of propaganda espousing the virtues of a high-protein diet. Milk builds strong bones and meat makes muscle, we were taught. Protein was eventually elevated to the status of supernutrient, the kingpin of a balanced diet, while vegetarians were portrayed as glassy-eyed zombies wasting away in San Francisco flophouses.

Those days are long gone. Nutritionists and dietitians have gradually, if somewhat grudgingly, conceded that protein requirements have been grossly overestimated and that the average American gets more than enough protein in the typical diet—in some cases, an excess of protein that strains the kidneys and acidifies the blood.

Protein is used by the body for construction, as opposed to being used for energy and maintenance. The amount of food used for body construction versus that used for energy stands at a ratio of about 1 to 7; therefore, the diet should reflect these general proportions of protein to carbohydrate intake. Nutritionists and the U.S. government have publicly recognized that meat and dairy products are no longer considered the revered cornerstones of the American diet, and it has been almost universally conceded that most people can survive quite well on a meat-free diet. Many respected researchers, nutritionists, and medical practitioners advocate a meat-free diet. Dr. T. Colin Campbell, one of the codirectors of the China Diet and Health Project, notes: "The closer we get to an all-plant diet, the better off we are. . . . Even small amounts of animal protein appear to be harmful for some people."

Ounce for ounce, bean products—such as tofu, tempeh, and soy milk—have about the same amount of protein as animal products, and grains have about half as much. Grains and legumes are equal, and often superior, to meats in terms of percentage of calories from protein compared with fat (Table 5).

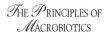

Table 5
PROTEIN, FAT, AND CALORIES IN GRAINS, LEGUMES, MEATS, AND FISH

FOOD	PROTEIN (GRAMS)	FAT (GRAMS)	CALORIES
Grains (1 cup cooked)			
Wild rice	9.7	1	200
Bulghur wheat	8.7	1	207
Oatmeal	6.6	2	156
Millet	6.3	2	210
Brown rice	4.9	1.6	218
Corn grits	3.5	<1	146
Legumes (1 cup cooked)			
Black beans	18.2	1.4	226
Lentils	17.9	<1	231
Kidney beans	16.2	<1	219
Split peas	16.4	<1	231
Lima beans	14.7	<1	217
Navy beans	15.8	1	259
Garbanzo beans	14.5	4	269
Meats/Fish (4 ounces cooked)			
Hamburger (broiled)	24.1	19	289
Lamb, leg (roasted)	21.6	17.4	256
Bacon (fried)	34.5	52.6	624
Chicken, light meat (broiled)	31.1	13.6	253
Turkey, light meat (broiled)	31.7	9.5	225
Rockfish	26.8	2.3	143
Haddock	25.5	1.2	121
Shrimp	23.4	1.2	112

Supplementation: Vitamins and More

Some controversy continues over the necessity of vitamin, mineral, and other nutritional supplementation in the daily diet. Many maintain that if an individual consumes a balanced, varied diet consisting of whole, natural foods, he or she should obtain all the necessary nutrients. Not so, say others—sadly enough, life just isn't that simple any more. Reasons and rationales for supplementation abound, given the many drastic changes in our social, cultural, and nutritional development.

Depleted Soil

Over the past several decades, soil in the major agricultural areas of the United States has been drastically depleted of many essential nutrients. These nutrients are lost to the crops that grow in the soil as well as to the livestock that feed upon it. The net result is that the food Americans consume does not contain what it should if grown under normal circumstances.

Transit Time and Storage

Although the ideal is to eat foods grown locally and regionally, the reality is that most people consume foods that are transported

When vegetarianism came into its heyday in the late 1960s, the angst and anxiety over obtaining adequate protein in a meat-free diet was addressed by the food-combining, or complementary-proteins, theory, which was widely espoused in the early 1970s. The complementary-proteins practice held that in order for one to obtain the necessary and optimal amount of protein, foods with complementary amino acids had to be consumed at the same meal. In other words, grains, which are high in certain amino acids but low in others, had to be consumed with beans, which are high in those amino acids lacking in grains. This led to rigorous and often impractical machinations of meal plans, as scores of would-be vegetarians struggled to make sure the grams of lysine in their bowls of beans were adequately complemented by the appropriate amount of tryptophan. Subsequent research has refuted that theory, and modern nutritionists now believe that complementary proteins must be consumed only during the course of a two- to three-day period—or even over a period as long as a week—rather than within a twenty-four-hour period.

There are additional compelling reasons for avoiding meat, not the least of which is the high amount of saturated fats in red meat, dairy products, and unskinned poultry. Saturated fats have been implicated in an increased risk of cancer, heart disease, and obesity and in a variety of other health ailments. Meat is difficult to digest: It decomposes as soon as it is killed and continues to putrefy in the stomach and digestive tract, requiring about four to five hours to be digested and absorbed in the intestines—compared with grains and vegetables, which require about two hours. Toxins released from meat during the digestive process accumulate in the organs, especially the liver and kidneys.

Certain ideological and moral mandates necessitated the exclusion of meat from the traditional macrobiotic diet. According to macrobiotic principles as put forth by George Ohsawa, vegetarians tend to be more calm, more patient, and less fatigued, while those who eat meat or meat products tend to be aggressive, egocentric, lazy, and vulnerable to disease. An old and widely held macrobiotic maxim holds that, of our thirty-two teeth, twenty are appropriate for grinding grain products, eight for chewing vegetables, and four for chewing meats—thereby establishing the "proper" proportion of these three nutritional elements in the diet.

Remember, however, that a macrobiotic diet is not necessarily vegetarian—indeed, the traditional macrobiotic diet includes fish, and some schools of practice allow small amounts of dairy and even some meats, based on climate, season, and individual physiological differences. Macrobiotic maxims encourage the consumption of flesh and animal products in their least altered states—that is, animals that are lower on the food chain, such as fish, and those that have undergone as little adulteration as possible.

This book, however, is based on a meat- and dairy-free diet, allowing only a small amount of fresh fish, mainly because of the plethora of hormones, additives, antibiotics, and other unnecessary and often harmful substances in commercially raised meats. The founders of the traditional macrobiotic diet could hardly have predicted these modern alterations.

A note here on vitamin B_{12}: When macrobiotic and vegetarian—especially vegan—diets began to grow in popularity, doctors and nutritionists cautioned followers of these regimens about vitamin B_{12} deficiencies, maintaining that vegetable sources of B_{12} do not exist. Other schools of thought have claimed that B_{12} is present in sea vegetables, spirulina, chlorella, tempeh, miso, and other fermented foods. Proponents of the vegan and macrobiotic diets hold that bacteria growing on fermented vegetarian foods, such as tempeh and miso, yield significant quantities of the vitamin.

A 1977 study by microbiologists from Cornell University at the Institute of Food Sciences in Geneva, New York, showed that one 3.5-ounce serving of Indonesian tempeh contained enough vitamin B_{12} to satisfy the Recommended Daily Allowance (RDA) set by the National Academy of Sciences, and independent research by tempeh companies following on the heels of these findings revealed significant levels of B_{12} in tempeh. However, later research found only trace amounts of B_{12} in dozens of samples of tempeh and miso, but significant levels of B_{12} were found in some sea vegetables and in spirulina. Another study yielded similar results: In a test of more than forty macrobiotic foods, only sea vegetables and spirulina contained B_{12}; the highest amounts were found in nori, kombu, and wakame. The samples of tempeh, miso, and tamari that were tested did not contain B_{12}. Some hypothesize that B_{12} is no longer contained in tempeh because of modern sanitation measures—tempeh is made from a mold that grows on fermented soybeans, and B_{12} comes not from the mold itself but rather from bacteria that grows on the mold. Indonesian tempeh, by contrast, has been found to contain appreciable levels of B_{12} because of poor sanitation measures in the region.

While the findings regarding tempeh and miso are somewhat discouraging, fish and sea vegetables—staples in the macrobiotic diet—do contain appreciable levels of B_{12}. A study published in the *American Journal of Clinical Nutrition* in 1988 found that macrobiotic and vegetarian mothers were able to obtain adequate amounts of dietary vitamin B_{12} by consuming sea vegetables. The body requires less B_{12} than any other vitamin, and it is remarkably efficient at storing B_{12}—some research indicates that it may take as long as twenty or thirty years to deplete the body's stores of the vitamin.

To be on the safe side, eat fish two to three times a week, consume sea vegetables daily, and take a high-quality vitamin B_{12} supplement if you're concerned about your B_{12} intake. (For more on supplementation issues, see sidebar on pages 28–31.)

and stored over a period of several days—and often more than a week—after they've been harvested. This transit and storage time allows for the depletion of vitamins and valuable enzymes.

Processing

Food technology made fantastic strides with the coming of the Industrial Revolution. Unfortunately, some of this technology has resulted in a substantial loss of nutrients. Processing of foods strips away vitamins, minerals, and trace elements. For example, when whole-wheat kernels are refined to make white flour, 83 percent of the nutrients in the wheat are lost. This is not an unusual example of the kind of nutrient loss that occurs with food processing.

Cooking

While cooking is necessary in the preparation of most foods, it depletes certain nutrients, especially if done improperly. For example, vitamins A, C, B_1, B_2, B_6, B_{12}, and D; folic acid; and pantothenic acid are unstable when subjected to heat. When foods containing these nutrients are cooked, vitamins can be lost. Minerals are also lost, although in lesser quantities.

DAIRY DILEMMAS

Numerous would-be vegetarians who earnestly attempt to abstain from flesh often turn to alternative sources of protein, increasing the amount of milk and cheese in their diets. At the risk of disillusioning those who are loath to relinquish their daily dairy fix, here's the bitter truth: excessive consumption of milk and other dairy products may be just as detrimental to overall health as meat, if not more so. The most recent and compelling reason for eschewing dairy is the approval by the Food and Drug Administration (FDA) of the use of genetically engineered hormones to boost milk production in cows. Consumers have no practical way of knowing whether dairy products on supermarket shelves contain bovine growth hormone (BGH), also known as BST or rBGH. The FDA does not currently require producers of milk and other dairy products to indicate on labeling that the products were made from the milk of cows treated with BGH. While the FDA maintains that growth hormones are safe and cause no side effects in humans, the use of BGH has been linked to an increase in mastitis, an infectious disease that causes inflammation of a cow's udders and requires treatment with antibiotics, which eventually find their way into the milk supply.

Other opponents of BGH point out that the federal government has been consistently and egregiously lacking in its efforts to adequately test milk for drug residues. The FDA estimates that in 1991 more than 170 million gallons of milk were discarded because of unsafe levels of drug residues. According to a General Accounting Office report released in 1993, tests that identified tainted milk were conducted for only four of the eighty-two possibly dangerous drugs used on dairy cows. If the FDA cannot guarantee safe levels of any drug residue in milk, how can it ensure that BGH is safe and that the consequent increase in antibiotic use will be detected?

A more serious health concern involves the close relationship between BGH and another hormone called insulinlike growth factor-1 (IGF-1). BGH causes an increase in the concentration of IGF-1 in cows' milk, according to a 1990 FDA report entitled *Bovine Growth Hormone: Human Food Safety Evaluation*. IGF-1 controls the body's response to growth hormones and has "acute metabolic and long-term, growth-promoting effects," according to the report. In addition, IGF-1 can cause acromegaly (an enlargement of the hands, feet, nose, and chin), glucose intolerance and hypertension, and has been linked to cancers and tumor growth.

There are numerous additionally compelling reasons for avoiding dairy products. Most studies have shown that between 50 and 90 percent of the world's population are lactose intolerant, meaning that they lack the necessary enzymes to digest dairy products, and that milk and milk products are generally inappropriate for human consumption. Casein, the protein in dairy, is extremely difficult for the body to assimilate and tends to cause excessive mucus in the body and hypersensitivity to allergens.

In addition, a number of different types of cancers have been related to high dairy consumption. One study published in the *Journal of the National Cancer Institute* in 1986 found an increased risk—between 1.5 and 1.8 percent higher—for breast cancer among women who consumed dairy products on a daily basis. In 1989 Harvard University researchers estimated that women who consume large amounts of yogurt and cottage cheese increase their risk of ovarian cancer as much as three times. The researchers believed that lactose, rather than fat content, was the key dietary variable for ovarian cancer.

Many women are concerned about excluding dairy from their diets for fear of not getting enough calcium, especially in light of the concern about the risk of osteoporosis. The body requires a balance of phosphorus and calcium, with a higher ratio of phosphorus to calcium, and dairy products are unable to provide that balance. High protein consumption has been linked to osteoporosis, and studies have shown that excess proteins actually increase the loss of calcium in the urine. It's a simple fallacy that the average person needs to consume dairy to ensure adequate calcium in the daily diet. One cup of turnip or collard greens contains about as much calcium as one cup of milk, and one three-ounce serving of tempeh contains about half as much (Table 6). In addition, sea vegetables are a valuable nondairy source of calcium, and sesame seeds have an ideal ratio of phosphorus to calcium.

Chemical Additives

Countless chemicals are used in processed foods, including artificial colors, flavors, preservatives, and sweeteners. Many of these chemicals are harmful, some are carcinogenic, and all force the body to use its antioxidant nutrients more quickly than it otherwise would to ward off the deleterious effects of the consumption of these chemical agents.

Biochemical Individuality

Each person is chemically unique, requiring a peculiar amount of nutrients. While some individuals require little of certain nutrients, other individuals may require enormous amounts. No two bodies are the same, and no two people's nutritional requirements are the same.

Other Factors

Environmental pollution, radiation, and other factors, such as the use of fluorescent lights, can also lead to a variety of health complications, many of which are related to nutrition. These factors can contribute to deficiencies of several nutrients.

can easily and rapidly lead to nutritional deficiency.

Table 6
COMPARISON OF CALCIUM CONTENT

Collard greens (1 cup)	290 mg
Milk (1 cup)	288 mg
Yogurt (1 cup)	272 mg
Turnip greens (1 cup)	252 mg
Mustard greens (1 cup)	194 mg
Kale (1 cup)	148 mg
Broccoli (1 cup)	136 mg
Hijiki, cooked ($^1/_4$ cup)	153 mg
Tempeh (3 ounces)	129 mg
Wakame ($^1/_4$ cup)	130 mg

3

MORE ON MACRO
Basic Principles and Modern Practices

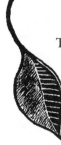

THE TRADITIONAL MACROBIOTIC DIET encompasses many principles, which you may or may not choose to follow on a strict basis. Try to incorporate as many of these principles as are practical for your lifestyle and level of commitment, but especially follow the principles for the purchase and consumption of organic foods. They're all valid, meaningful practices that will further maintain your diet and enhance your overall health.

EATING CLOSE TO HOME: REGIONAL DIETS AND ORGANIC FOOD

One of the principles of macrobiotics is based on the general practice of consuming locally grown foods—foods that are produced within a 500-mile radius of your home. In Japanese, the practice is known as the law of *Shi Do Fu Ji*, or "body and soil are one." The rationale behind this practice is that one who consumes locally grown foods eats in accordance with his or her personal climate and atmosphere and helps to maintain the natural order of the environment as a whole.

Tropical fruits and vegetables are thought to be excessively cooling, so unless you live in a truly balmy climate, they are generally considered inappropriate for a traditional macrobiotic diet. In addition, foods that are grown in other regions must be transported and, as a result, may be treated with preservatives to extend their shelf life and retard spoilage. One not insignificant result of this practice is that it translates into an enormous impact on the environment in terms of costs of production, refrigeration, transportation, and long-term soil degradation.

The importance of consuming organic foods cannot be overemphasized, even for those who choose not to follow a macrobiotic diet. Organic agriculture is defined as a long-term, systematic approach to growing food, with the ultimate goals of halting degradation of the soil and the environment, moving toward natural methods of agriculture, and reestablishing the balance of the environment. In practical terms, following organic growing practices means that growers cease using artificial chemicals and fertilizers, create alternatives to high-tech agricultural practices, implement techniques such as integrated pest management and integrated nutrient management, and generally apply a minimum of external influences (artificial chemicals, pesticides, and fertilizers) in order to allow the earth and soil to return to a state of balance in which agriculture can be indefinitely sustained.

Consider the environmental cost of pesticides and the hidden prices related to foods grown by conventional farming methods. In 1992 a Cornell University researcher estimated that the indirect costs of pesticide use totaled more than $8 billion a year, with $787 million related to public health impacts, $520 million to loss of natural pest enemies, $2.1 billion to bird losses, $1.8 billion to groundwater contamination, $1.4 billion to crop pesticide resistance, $942 million to crop losses, and a combined total of $574 million in costs related to domestic animal deaths and contamination, honeybee and pollination losses, fishery losses, and the price of formulating and enforcing government regulations to prevent damage.

A recent report by the Worldwatch Institute in Washington, D.C., found that the population increase, from 2.6 billion to 5.5 billion since 1950, has begun to outstrip the carrying capacity of biological support systems and the ability of natural systems to absorb waste without being damaged. And if you happen to have children, consider this: The National Academy of Sciences released a report in June 1993 entitled *Pesticides in the Diets of Infants and Children,* which estimated that the average American child exceeds the Environmental Protection Agency's (EPA's) lifetime risk standard from pesticides in food by his or her first birthday. These findings were based on cancer risks from eight pesticides in twenty fruits and vegetables. According to the report, levels of farm chemical residues in foods "could be sufficiently high to produce symptoms of acute pesticide poisoning" for some children. A subsequent report in 1993 by the Environmental Working Group, a Washington, D.C.–based consumer organization, concluded that "the average child exceeds the EPA lifetime one-in-one-million risk standard by his or her first birthday." The major conclusion of the report was that "the federal government's decision-making process for pesticides does not pay sufficient attention to the protection of human health, especially the health of infants and children."

Organic food consumption is hardly a passing fad. Sales of organic products increased 25 percent in 1991, and in 1992 organic sales topped $1.5 billion. A recent study of consumers showed an increasing awareness of and preference for organic foods. *The Organic Trend Report: Shoppers and Products,* released in September 1993 by HealthFocus Inc., surveyed more than 1,000 Americans and found that most consumers know what organic foods are and are aware of their health benefits; 14 percent of American shoppers use organic produce at least once a week. The study also found that the introduction of organic products has expanded into forty-six different food categories since 1988, and the greatest growth has been in grains and vegetable protein products.

ADJUSTING FOR VARIOUS FACTORS: YOUR BODY, YOUR ENVIRONMENT

While the macrobiotic diet incorporates certain caveats regarding seemingly strict adherence to a prescribed diet with a formula of foods, it does not overlook the importance of various factors such as personal physiological differences, age, activity level, seasonal adjustments, and climatic variables. Just as yin and yang are balanced at each meal, they also must be balanced within the larger picture of who the individual is and where he or she lives.

Your Body: What You Live In

No two bodies are the same. Size, age, activity level, and genetic constitution all play a part in the balance of yin and yang and the choices of food. Saigon Ishizuku and George Ohsawa believed that differences in body makeup, such as color of skin, weight, size, speed of growth, strength, longevity, susceptibility to sickness, voice, and memory, are dependent on environmental conditions and the balance of potassium and salt foods in the diet—a concept later refined by Ohsawa to reflect the balance of yin and yang foods in the diet.

According to the principles of yin and yang, yin tends to be more female, yang more male. Men are presumed by macrobiotic maxims to have hardier, stronger constitutions and physical builds than women and, consequently, require more yang influences in terms of food selection and preparation. Richer, more dense foods, root vegetables, protein foods, slightly heavier seasonings, more oils, and longer, warmer cooking methods, as used when baking and frying or making casseroles, are generally recommended for men. By the same token, raw foods, fruits, and sweets should be reduced.

Women, on the other hand, are presumed under the macrobiotic philosophy to have more delicate constitutions, thus requiring more yin, or lighter, food types and cooking methods. More leafy green vegetables and shorter cooking times are prescribed for women, and fruits, sweets, and raw foods can be consumed slightly more often. Protein intake, especially the consumption of meat and fish, should be lower, seasonings should be lighter, and the use of oils should be slightly reduced.

All of this, of course, presumes a general condition of overall health and does not take into account such factors as size, age, general constitution, and activity level. A young female triathelete with a larger-than-average body build and a strong constitution can tend toward more yang foods than a sedentary, older female with a weaker constitution. In addition, women have certain special needs that men do not. Excessively yin or yang foods, such as animal protein, salt, and sweets, should be reduced during the menstrual cycle to help prevent cramps, bloating, headaches, and other difficulties. In general, if you're a woman and you have painful or problematic menstrual cycles, try to be especially vigilant about making your diet fall toward the middle range of foods on the yin/yang scale, tending toward grains, a balance of leafy green and root vegetables, small portions of legumes, less oil and condiments, and moderate cooking methods.

People who are extremely active can easily accommodate more yang influences in their diets—they can increase protein intake, eat more root vegetables, use slightly more oils and seasonings, and use stronger cooking methods such as frying and baking. These adjustments are necessary for strengthening and maintaining energy levels. People who have sedentary jobs and lower activity levels require more yin influences in the diet: Protein and stimulating foods should be reduced, and the total quantity of foods consumed should be less than that required by a highly active person. People whose jobs or professions require extended periods of intense mental, rather than physical, activity are advised to add more sea vegetables to their daily diets to help balance and stabilize thoughts and emotions.

According to the macrobiotic philosophy, certain adjustments to the diet are assumed to be necessary for spiritual inclinations and levels of development. During times of excessive stress and tension, or if you wish to further your spiritual development through meditation and prayer, the macrobiotic maxim advises adhering to a diet composed strictly of whole grains and vegetables and avoiding all animal products, strong condiments, and spices (spices are strong stimulants, and the Japanese traditionally believed spices created mental confusion and impeded clear and calm thinking). The amount of food consumed should be reduced, and the diet should consist of brown rice, miso soup, sea vegetables, and a small amount of land vegetables and legumes. Millet, barley, and corn are also thought to help meditation practices.

Regular fasting for short periods of time on brown rice and liquids is traditional macrobiotic practice. Traditional macrobiotic maxims hold that brown rice fasts can be continued for as long as ten days, but in modern practices a fast for this length of time should be attempted only with nutritional and medical supervision. A one- or two-day brown-rice fast with adequate liquid intake can generally be undertaken safely and comfortably, unless you have some sort of medical disorder.

Your Environment: Where You Live

The principles of yin and yang are based on the concept that the universe consists of constant change. As the seasons change, so do our needs. Differences in diet according to season are often significant. The principal foods and condiments used, and the methods by which they are prepared, differ dramatically from warm to cold seasons. In late spring and summer, more yin, or cooling, foods should be consumed to offset the yang, or heating, factors of the climate. In cold-weather months, more yang foods should be incorporated for their warming influences.

In addition, climatic differences must be taken into account. If you live in the tropics, your dietary needs will be very different from those of people who live in Arctic climates. Generally, people who live in colder climates require a slightly more yang influence in the diet, while those who live in warm climates may use more yin foods.

WINTER

In most cases and climates, winter is a time of cold, damp influences. To offset these external influences and help the body better adjust to the environment, consume foods that are more warming and dense. Keep raw foods to a minimum and emphasize cooked foods such as rich stews, hearty casseroles, and baked dishes. Bean products and root vegetables in particular are warming and strengthening and can help the body adjust to cold weather. Soups should be consumed at least once a day. Protein foods may be increased. Seasonings can be moderately stronger, the amount of oil used in cooking may be increased slightly, and liquid consumption should be reduced.

SPRING

According to macrobiotic philosophy, the energy within the body becomes less contracted and more expansive as the weather warms and snows begin to thaw. The body begins to reach upward and outward as we become more active and spend more time outside. Accordingly, the diet should focus on

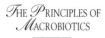

foods that tend to be more upward and expansive. Root vegetables and protein foods are gradually lessened, and leafy greens play a more prominent role in the diet. Cooking and preparation tends to be quicker and lighter, and seasonings and oils are slightly decreased.

SUMMER

As the weather continues to warm, more cooling influences are necessary in the diet. Vegetables with a more yin, or expansive, energy—leafy greens, sprouts, lettuces, corn, cucumber, and squash—should be used along with small amounts of fruit. Heavy protein foods are minimized, and tofu, which has a mild cooling influence, can be emphasized as a source of protein. Foods should be cooked lightly, with little oil and a decreased amount of seasonings, and some dishes may be served slightly chilled. Liquid consumption should also be increased.

FALL

As autumn approaches, the body begins to draw in once again, contracting in preparation for the onset of winter. More warming vegetables—winter squashes, turnips, cabbage, and root vegetables—can be introduced into the diet, and soups and stews may be used more often. Cooking methods again become longer, and oils and seasonings—especially miso and shoyu—may be gradually increased. Raw foods and fruits should be decreased. Protein foods, especially beans and tempeh, may be increased.

TREASURES FROM THE SEA

One of the most initially unfamiliar aspects of the macrobiotic diet is the use of sea vegetables. In the standard macrobiotic diet, sea vegetables constitute about 5 percent of the daily regimen. If they're not properly prepared, sea vegetables are hardly appealing, and they generally resemble aquarium fillers. With appropriate aesthetic adaptations, however, it's quite simple to incorporate seaweed into a modern diet. One-third ounce (dry weight) of sea vegetables daily is recommended on the macrobiotic diet, and this addition can be easily accomplished. Toss a handful of wakame, hijiki, or arame in salads, soups, or cooked grains, or crumble them over cooked vegetables. Add dulse to soups and stews, use leftover rice and vegetables wrapped in nori for vegetarian sushi, and prepare soup and sauce stocks with kombu (more details are included in the recipes that follow).

Over the years, sea vegetables have been used for a variety of purposes—as everything from fertilizer and a source of salt to stabilizing agents and emulsifiers in cosmetics and processed foods. Oriental texts and tales tell of Japanese women who subsisted mainly on seaweed and grew long, strong, thick hair, which they lopped off and sold to be fashioned into durable cords for hauling stone blocks across the fields and mountains to Kyoto. Hundreds of years later, some of those heavy ropes of hair still hang in the Honganji Cathedral near the center of the city.

Although getting used to the taste of sea vegetables may take ardent effort on the part of your palate, you can learn to appreciate their rich, tangy flavor. Start with milder seaweeds, such as arame, and work your way up to the stronger ones, like hijiki and kombu. If nothing else, the extraordinarily high nutritional value of seaweeds should convince you to make them a portion of your daily diet. They're rich in calcium, iron, vitamins, minerals, and trace minerals, including selenium, zinc, copper, and molybdenum; they contain substantial levels of potassium, which aids in elimination and regulates the heartbeat; and they are rich in calcium and phosphorus, which are important for blood coagulation, building bones and teeth, activating enzymes and normalizing metabolism, and aiding in the transport of fatty acids.

Sea vegetables are highly alkaline, helping to balance acidic blood conditions, and they are believed to have blood-cleansing and -strengthening properties. Dulse is especially high in magnesium, which strengthens nerves, tones muscle, and activates enzymes in carbohydrate metabolism, and in iron, which aids in hemoglobin, bone, brain, and muscle-tissue formation. Kelp is high in iodine, which aids in the oxidation of fats and proteins and stimulates circulation. (See pages 47–49 for a description of the types of sea vegetables.)

GARNISHES, CONDIMENTS, AND SEASONINGS

The traditional macrobiotic diet uses various kinds of often unfamiliar but highly flavorful supplementary foods for health and aesthetic purposes. A pinch of gomashio greatly enhances the flavor of grains; a small pile of peach-colored pickled ginger on the side of a dish adds aesthetic value and aids digestion; a little grated daikon helps balance fish and high-protein meals. Most of the following ingredients can be found in Oriental food markets and some natural-products stores. Experiment freely with these garnishes, condiments, and seasonings—you'll find limitless ways to use them creatively.

Garnishes

Most garnishes are either pickled or raw grated foods, frequently used to balance the yang effects of meat meals. Daikon root is a slightly peppery, pale-white garnish that is generally served grated. It adds a fresh appearance and taste, especially to fish and heavy noodle meals. Grated horseradish and grated radish are used in much the same way as daikon root. Nori and other seaweeds can be lightly toasted and either cut into strips or crumbled and sprinkled on top of soups, grain dishes, salads, and vegetables. Finely chopped scallions are often floated on top of miso soup to brighten the appearance and to add flavor, and they may be included in noodle dishes or sprinkled on tempeh and fish. Wasabi—a pungent green horseradish—and red or black pepper, sometimes mixed with sesame seeds, are also used in small quantities.

Condiments

One of the most frequently used condiments in macrobiotic cooking is gomashio, a balanced mixture of roasted, lightly crushed sesame seeds and unrefined sea salt. It's a versatile, healthy substitute for salt that should be a staple in your kitchen. Use it as you would salt, especially on grains, noodle dishes, and cooked vegetables. Tekka is a pungent, highly concentrated mixture of cooked vegetables in the form of a dark brown powder. Sprinkle it lightly on cooked vegetables and grains instead of salt for a rich, hearty flavor. Miso, another staple in the macrobiotic kitchen, is a thick paste with a rich, slightly sweet taste and is used as a condiment or seasoning. Miso is made from fermented soybeans mixed with other grains, sea salt, and koji, an enzyme starter that facilitates the fermentation process.

Other macrobiotic condiments include pickled ginger, used to aid digestion and impart warming energy; umeboshi plum, a sour, pickled Japanese plum served sliced or whole as a side dish or used in paste form in cooking; roasted sea vegetables, ground and sometimes combined with sesame seeds and a small amount of roasted sea salt; shiso or beefsteak leaves, generally chopped and used with grains and soups; and mustard, often used to balance seafood dishes.

Seasonings

Seasonings in macrobiotic cooking are carefully selected, with balance and moderation in mind. Salt, the most commonly used seasoning in most American households, has its place in macrobiotic cooking as well—the main difference lies in the type and quantity used. Macrobiotics eschews the use of the typical highly processed and refined white table salt common to the modern diet in favor of roasted, unrefined sea salt, which is rich in trace minerals. Even then, much smaller quantities are generally used. Salt is used in cooking, rather than sprinkled on foods, and it is generally recommended that salt be cooked in foods for a minimum of fifteen to twenty minutes to allow the salt to combine with nutrients in the foods and become more easily assimilated by the body. (If you're cocking your eyebrows with consternation and mistrust at the mere suggestion that you sully your diet with salt, see "Using Salt," page 40–41.)

Shoyu, similar to soy sauce, is a commonly used substitute for salt in macrobiotic cooking. Shoyu is a high-quality fermented liquid made from soybeans, wheat, water, and unrefined sea salt and contains no additives or artificial ingredients—it is quite different from the soy sauce found on most supermarket shelves, which typically contains monosodium glutamate (MSG), caramel coloring, sugar, refined salt, preservatives, and other additives. Shoyu is also known as tamari, the term Ohsawa used to differentiate true shoyu from commercially prepared soy sauce. Originally, tamari was the name of the liquid by-product of miso production and contained no wheat or grain products. When the terms became confused, "real tamari" and "genuine tamari" were introduced. In general, shoyu contains wheat and tamari does not.

USING SALT

The orthodox medical community and mainstream media have proffered and promulgated a widespread and sweeping indictment of salt, linking it to hypertension, heart disease, and other health horrors. While somewhat simplified, theirs is a concern not without validity. Since the typical modern diet consists of an inordinate quantity of processed foods—including everything from Cheetos to Cheerios—most Americans get more than their share of salt without using it in cooking or adding it to a dish as a seasoning. According to macrobiotic philosophy, salt is a beneficial, alkaline-forming food, and, without the proper amount, the body's immunity is decreased and health is compromised. If your diet is composed of whole, unprocessed foods and little or no animal protein, it's possible that you may not get enough sodium to maintain an alkaline condition of the body fluids or the proper potassium and sodium ratio between intercellular and intracellular fluids if you eschew salt.

Salt has received more negative publicity than almost any other dietary element, but this much-maligned mineral has numerous crucial biological functions. It's true that diets high in salt have been linked to hypertension, but most people with high blood pressure also have contributing dietary and lifestyle factors—including excessive consumption of animal products, processed products, and high-fat foods—which must be taken into consideration. Sodium and chlorides remain outside the body's cells, and potassium and phosphates remain inside the cells, maintaining a balance to ensure the proper functioning of cells and organs. Sodium is crucial to the digestive process, aiding in the production of bile, stimulating the peristaltic movement of the digestive tract, affecting muscle strength, and aiding in the production of hydrochloric acid. Diets excessively low in salt can lead to malaise, cold hands and feet, and leg cramps.

That's the Western view. In more macrobiotic terms, potassium is yin, sodium is yang, and both elements must be present in the body, in a recommended ratio of 5–7 parts potassium to 1 part sodium, for optimal health. The key is to achieve a balance between potassium and sodium—*balance* being the operative term. According to Saigon Ishizuku's teachings, most of the body is composed of inorganic nutrients, which control the workings of the organs, metabolic activity, and proper functioning of the nervous system. His theory held that the most important inorganic minerals in the body are potassium and sodium, both of which are salts. Potassium and sodium are antagonistic in the body and must be consumed in the proper proportions for optimal health.

It's difficult for the body to assimilate salt, which, if introduced in large amounts into the intercellular channels, does not modify levels of intracellular potassium to create a desirable ratio or balance. Raw table salt changes the sodium content of the blood and disturbs heart functioning, and it passes through the alimentary canal and acts as a stimulant. In the macrobiotic diet, salt is used in cooking or in condiment form, combined with oil or organic matter, so that it can be properly absorbed without excessively stimulating the nervous system or the kidneys. Food is cooked for at least twenty minutes after the addition of salt to ensure that the sodium combines with nutrients and organic matter in the food, allowing for proper absorption and bioavailability.

In addition, the refined table salt most Americans use lacks minerals and trace minerals that help enzymatic action crucial for digestion and metabolism. Hence the reliance in the macrobiotic diet on tekka, miso, gomashio, and tamari, which also contain potassium to balance their sodium content.

SAVORING SOUPS

It is the Japanese custom to start the day with a bowl of clear broth or miso soup to energize and gently awaken the digestive system after several hours of fasting. In the United States, soup for breakfast is a decidedly acquired taste—but it can, indeed, be acquired, and it's a healthy alternative to Danishes and doughnuts. Miso soup is an ideal way to start the day, warming and energizing the body, and it's a good source of protein and B vitamins, contains friendly bacteria that can help replenish intestinal flora, aids in digestion, and is said to strengthen the blood. In warm weather, it can be taken at room temperature. All that aside, it's fast, easy, and absurdly convenient.

One frequently used method of preparing soups is called layering, a technique in which the most yin ingredients—onions, celery, and mushrooms, for example—are placed on the bottom of the pot, where they'll acquire the most heat and yang energy during cooking. More yang vegetables—carrots, burdock, and various root vegetables—comprise the next layers, along with grains (some grains, like barley and rice, are cooked first, since they require longer cooking times than most vegetables). Leafy greens are added last, during the final stages of cooking. The layering theory holds that yin flavors expand upward during cooking and yang flavors, conversely, sink, allowing the flavors to blend and harmonize without excessive mixing and stirring. A pinch of sea salt is sprinkled on the top of the layers of ingredients, and water is added by pouring it carefully down the sides of the pot before and during cooking as needed, to avoid disturbing the layers.

Two bowls of soup a day are recommended in the macrobiotic diet. If you start your day with a light miso broth, you might add a bowl of richer miso- or kombu-based stock with noodles and vegetables as an appetizer or light lunch. Or make a hearty soup with barley, rice, or other grains; tempeh or tofu; and a variety of vegetables. Thickening agents like kuzu, arrowroot, and flour make creamy and rich stews.

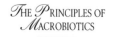

PART TWO

THE PRACTICE OF MACROBIOTICS

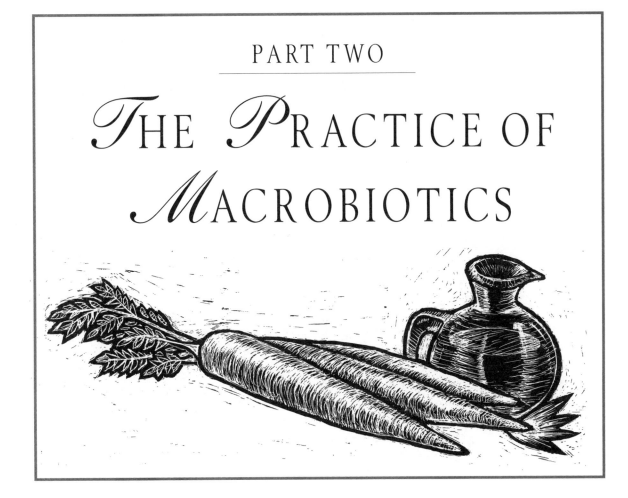

4

GETTING STARTED
Stocking the Kitchen

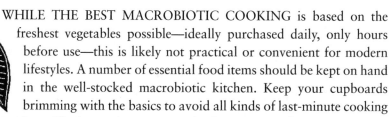

WHILE THE BEST MACROBIOTIC COOKING is based on the freshest vegetables possible—ideally purchased daily, only hours before use—this is likely not practical or convenient for modern lifestyles. A number of essential food items should be kept on hand in the well-stocked macrobiotic kitchen. Keep your cupboards brimming with the basics to avoid all kinds of last-minute cooking crises—and you'll always have most of what you need to prepare any macrobiotic meal in a flash. (See also Appendix B: Grocery Shopping List.)

Most macrobiotic staples can be found in natural-products stores and Oriental markets. If you live in a large, metropolitan area, you'll likely be able to find many or most of these staples—including soy milk, miso, and organic produce—at your local supermarket, often at more competitive prices. Try making two stops on your shopping day—first at the natural-products store, then at the Oriental market to fill in the gaps. If you're having problems finding some of the ingredients listed in the sections above, check Appendix D: Mail-Order Guide and Resource List.

SEASONINGS, CONDIMENTS, AND SEA VEGETABLES

Many of the unique flavors and textures in macrobiotic cooking are dependent on a number of not-so-common ingredients, so there are several seasonings, condiments, and sea vegetables that should be part of a well-stocked kitchen. Most of these items can be purchased in your local natural-products store or in any Oriental market. If you shop in Oriental markets, check labels carefully—some products contain refined salt, sugar, monosodium glutamate (MSG), and artificial additives and preservatives.

Keep all of the following ingredients in glass containers with tight-fitting lids. Some foods, such as miso and tamari, should never be refrigerated, even though you may find them in the refrigerated section of your store. Miso and tamari may both be stored in a pantry or on a kitchen shelf. Sometimes a white film or coating may appear on the miso. It's harmless—just stir it back into the miso and use as you normally would.

Miso

Miso is a fermented condiment made from soybeans and other grains, with sea salt and koji, an enzyme starter. Oriental mythology holds that miso was a food bestowed upon humankind to ensure long life, health, and prosperity. The *Journal of Nutritional Sciences and Vitaminology* reported in early 1994 that miso may help prevent breast cancer and chronic kidney inflammation, possibly as a result of its high content of vitamin E and other antioxidants, including isoflavones and saponins. In addition, a University of Alabama cancer study found that animals fed miso and other fermented soy products had fewer tumors, more benign tumors, and a slower growth rate of malignancy than a control group of animals not fed these items. The researchers suggested that miso consumption may be a factor in the lower incidence of breast cancer in Japanese women, and they concluded that "organic compounds in fermented soybean-based foods may exert a chemoprotective effect."

Miso is available in many varieties and flavors including mugi miso, which contains barley; kome or rice miso; shiro, a sweeter white-rice miso; aka or red miso; natto miso, made from soybeans, grains, and ginger; hatcho miso, a thick, dry paste made from soybeans and koji; and soba miso, made from buckwheat. Miso contains living organisms and should be added during the last stage of cooking to preserve its nutritional value and prevent the destruction of valuable enzymes.

Unrefined Sea Salt

A staple in the macrobiotic kitchen, unrefined sea salt differs from the bleached and highly refined table salt generally found in American kitchens. It can generally be purchased in bulk in most natural-products stores. Store it in a glass container with a tight-fitting lid.

Gomashio

Gomashio can be used as a salt substitute and is an indispensable seasoning in macrobiotic cooking. It is made from unrefined sea salt and slightly crushed sesame seeds. Because the seeds are crushed, the oil is more volatile. Buy it in small quantities—the smallest jar available will generally last most families for at least a week.

Umeboshi Plums

An umeboshi plum is a type of Japanese apricot that is dried and pickled for at least six months. The plums have a tangy, salty taste and can be purchased whole or in paste form. The longer they age, the less tart and salty they become. Whole plums are generally preferable to the paste, since the nutrients become somewhat dissipated after they have been pureed.

Shoyu and Tamari

Shoyu and tamari are available at natural-products stores and are quite different from the soy sauces on the shelves at conventional grocery stores. Soy sauce generally contains sugar, refined salt, and caramel colorings and may have preservatives and MSG as well. Some confusion remains about the difference between shoyu and tamari. Shoyu is a fermented seasoning made from soybeans, wheat, water, and unrefined sea salt. *Tamari* is a derivation of the word for the liquid by-product of the miso fermentation process, and the seasoning does not contain wheat.

Wasabi

Green horseradish, a seasoning called wasabi, is found in powdered or paste form at most natural-products stores. The powder form is much more pungent and warming and is preferable to the paste. To prepare the powder for serving as a dip or in sauces, add a few drops of water to a tablespoon of the dried powder, and allow it to sit for about ten minutes to fully develop the flavor.

Tekka

Tekka is a highly concentrated seasoning used in very small amounts in macrobiotic cooking. It has a smoky, distinctive flavor and is made of burdock, carrots, hatcho miso, ginger, and lotus root cooked in heavy iron pots with dark sesame oil until it becomes a concentrated black powder. Tekka may be found at most natural-products stores or Oriental markets and should be stored, tightly sealed, in a glass container.

Vinegar

Vinegar comes in a variety of forms and flavors. The vinegars sold in most supermarkets, including white vinegar and wine vinegar, are generally not appropriate for macrobiotic cooking. Brown rice vinegar is most often used in macrobiotic cooking and can be found in natural-products stores and some supermarkets. Umeboshi vinegar, a byproduct of the umeboshi pickling process, is used on occasion.

Ginger

Fresh ginger is eminently preferable to the dried and powdered forms, which lack the warming energy of the root. Ginger may be purchased whole at almost any grocery or natural-products store and can be found pickled in plastic or foil containers at Oriental specialty stores. Store fresh ginger root in a cool, dry place and grate or mince as needed, refrigerating the rest of the root after it has been cut. Use pickled ginger as a garnish.

Sweeteners

Sweeteners are used in small amounts in macrobiotic cooking. The most commonly used forms are barley malt syrup, brown rice syrup, and mirin, a sweet winelike liquid made from fermented rice. Mirin should be purchased in small amounts and kept refrigerated. It's often available in bulk form at natural-products stores, as are barley malt syrup and brown rice syrup. Sweeteners cannot always be substituted in equal parts. In most recipes about twice as much brown rice syrup, barley malt syrup, and concentrated fruit juice sweetener is used as honey, maple syrup, or molasses; a slight reduction in liquid is required in the recipe when fruit juice, honey, and maple syrup are used.

Oils

The highly refined and processed oils sold in most supermarkets are unsuitable for the macrobiotic diet. Purchase oils in small quantities from a natural-products store, and buy only enough to last a week (many oils are available in natural-products stores in the bulk section at a substantial cost savings). The basic oils to keep on hand include toasted sesame oil, unrefined corn oil, sunflower oil, soybean oil, and olive oil. Keep them in a cupboard after opening, or if you won't be able to use them within a week, store them in the refrigerator to keep them from going rancid.

Sea Vegetables

A variety of sea vegetables should be kept on hand for all macrobiotic cooking needs. Arame, hijiki, kombu, wakame, and nori are the mainstays. Buy enough sea vegetables to last one week—you may need to experiment with the quantity you purchase to adjust to your tastes and personal needs. Buy sea vegetables from a reputable natural-products store, since some of them may be treated with alkaline chemical solutions, chlorine, and other bleaching agents. Sea vegetables are also available in flake or powder form, but these forms are generally inferior to the whole form. You can powder your own sea vegetables at home in a suribachi or with a mortar and pestle. Keep sea vegetables tightly sealed in glass containers or plastic bags in a dark, dry location. Wakame, arame, hijiki, and kombu should be rinsed well and soaked for three to five minutes, in just enough water to cover them, before cooking.

Sea vegetables are generally grouped into four categories, depending on their color: brown algae, red algae, green algae, and blue/green algae. The color of the sea vegetable depends on the depth at which it grows in the ocean, which consequently determines the amount of light it receives from the sun. The most commonly used seaweeds and their properties are discussed below.

ARAME
A brown algae with large, leaf-shaped fronds that become black and wiry after drying and shredding, arame is a delicate seaweed, with a slightly sweet taste and firm texture. It is one of the more palatable selections for those who are just becoming acquainted with seaweeds.

HIJIKI
Hijiki (or hiziki) is a brown algae that has short, needle-shaped fronds and is black in color when dried. It has a slightly nutty flavor and holds up well in soups, stews, and stir-fries. Hijiki also has the highest content of calcium and iron of the sea vegetables and is used in Japan to strengthen the bones, hair, and intestines and to rejuvenate and freshen skin.

KOMBU
Kombu is a brown algae most often used for stocks and soup broths. It is dark brownish or blackish green when dried and has long, broad fronds. It has a slightly stronger flavor than some of the other seaweeds. Kombu contains glutamic acid, which tenderizes and adds flavor to foods. It is used in cooking beans and grains to make them more tender and easier to digest, as well as to add flavor and shorten cooking time.

WAKAME
This brown algae turns a bright, almost transparent green during cooking or after soaking. Wakame has a slightly sweet flavor and is most often used in miso and other soups. It may be added to salads and grain dishes for color and flavor.

NORI
A red algae that grows with long, thin fronds but is generally chopped and dried into thin, rectangular sheets, nori has a milder taste and is the sea vegetable used to make sushi rolls. It can also be toasted and crumbled as a garnish or seasoning.

DULSE

Dulse is a red algae with a tangy and distinctive flavor. It is another ideal transitional sea vegetable and can be used in soups and baked dishes or crumbled onto grain dishes, cooked vegetables and salads.

AGAR-AGAR

Agar-agar (kanten) is a red algae whose fronds are exposed to intense sunlight to remove much of the flavor and color. It is then processed into flakes, powder, or bars. Agar-agar is generally dissolved in hot liquid and used as a thickening agent or gel for desserts, puddings, aspics, and other dishes.

SEA PALM

A green algae with small green fronds, sea palm is roasted and ground as a condiment. It can be used like kombu to tenderize vegetables, grains, and beans during cooking.

VEGETABLES AND FRUITS

An ideal practice is to buy fresh foods as often as possible. While a daily trip to the grocery store is inconvenient at best and supremely irritating at worst, there are ways to follow this maxim without lugging home paper bags brimming with Brussels sprouts and Belgian endive every night.

Vegetables

In general, root vegetables, including rutabagas, parsnips, carrots, turnips, burdock, and daikon, may be purchased weekly and stored in a cool, dark place. Most aboveground vegetables—broccoli, squash, green beans, cauliflower, and so on—can also be purchased on a weekly basis, as can greens such as kale, chard, and mustard greens. When planning your meals, try to use greens toward the beginning of the week, leaving the sturdier vegetables for later. Delicate leafy greens, lettuces, and sprouts should ideally be purchased the day you plan to use them, but this is by no means a hard and fast rule. To avoid more than two trips a week to the grocery store, try to schedule your meals to use the more delicate, highly perishable vegetables right after your shopping trips. Or make use of some of the boiled vegetable salads listed in the recipe section.

In traditional macrobiotic practices, all vegetables were stored in a root cellar, pantry, or other cool, dark place. Refrigeration was not always widely available, and macrobiotic principles hold that refrigeration, being cold and damp, imparts an excessive yin energy to foods. Thus, everything from rutabagas to kale was left unrefrigerated. If you have the space, location, and inclination, consider alternatives to refrigeration, as long as you don't live in an excessively warm climate. Root vegetables keep quite nicely out of the refrigerator. Limp or slightly wilted vegetables are suitable for soups, stews, and stir-fries, and they fare just fine when steamed, baked, or boiled as side dishes.

Never wash vegetables before storing—washing causes a loss of vitamins and minerals and makes the vegetables more likely to mold and soften. In addition, dirt or soil left on the vegetables will keep them fresh until you're ready to use them.

Fruits

While fruit is not a mainstay of the macrobiotic diet, certain temperate fruits, such as apples and pears, may be used several times a week. Tropical fruits, including mango, banana, and avocado, are strongly discouraged. Fruits should be organic, purchased whole rather than cut, fresh rather than frozen or canned. Temperate climate fruits should be stored in a cool, dark place rather than refrigerated, and melons and other highly perishable fruits should be kept refrigerated once cut. Have an assortment of dried fruits, such as apricots and raisins, on hand to liven up any number of dishes—toss a handful in salads, use them as desserts or side dishes, and add to leftover grains for breakfast cereals or cold salads. Dried fruits should be naturally dried—commercially dried fruits usually contain sulfur dioxide or methyl bromide.

PROTEIN FOODS

Tempeh, Tofu, and Seitan

Tempeh, tofu, and seitan should be kept on hand, since macrobiotic diets use them in small amounts on a daily basis. Tempeh keeps quite well in the refrigerator. You can buy several packages and freeze them; thaw them in the refrigerator the day before you plan to use them. Buy a variety of tempeh to use in different recipes—tempeh is available with quinoa, rice and other grains, sea vegetables, and a variety of legumes.

Tofu should be purchased on a weekly basis—buy both the firm and the silken variety. Both will keep for about a week after they've been opened. Store them in covered containers and change the water daily to keep them fresh. The silken variety can be blended with a variety of ingredients and seasonings for dressings and sandwich spreads, used to thicken soups and casseroles, blended with a small amount of nut butter and brown rice syrup as a dessert topping, or mixed with a little vinegar as a substitute for sour cream. Toward the end of the week, as firm tofu gets older, rinse it well, pat dry, and store in the freezer in a plastic bag. The day before you plan to use the tofu, let it thaw in the refrigerator, then squeeze out the excess moisture and crumble into soups and stir-fries. After freezing, the tofu will have a slightly yellowish color and a firmer, more meatlike texture that does well in hearty stews.

Seitan—a protein-rich, meatlike substance made from wheat gluten and cooked in tamari—keeps quite well for at least a week. It should be a staple in your kitchen for use in noodle dishes, stews, and casseroles and as a sandwich filling.

Milk Substitutes

Rice and soy milk should be kept on hand to use in a variety of recipes. Rice milk is lighter and slightly sweeter than soy milk, lending itself well to breakfast porridges and cereals. Soy milk is somewhat richer with a more distinctive, beany taste, and it works better in soups and sauces. Both come in a variety of flavors, with wide variances in fat content and ingredients, including added calcium, casein (milk protein), and sugar. Check the ingredients list and stick to the types made with organic rice and soybeans and those with the simplest ingredients. Purchase plain soy milk and vanilla-flavored rice milk for most uses.

Forget about the "lite" label on soy milk—it's generally a marketing ploy. In most cases, the product is light not because the soybeans are defatted but simply because the soy milk is diluted with water, thus diluting the nutrient content as well. Unless you want to pay for aseptically packaged water, make your own "light" soy milk at home. Buy the regular variety and dilute it with pure spring water. Store it covered and refrigerated in a glass container.

Cheese Substitutes

Rice, soy, and nut cheeses are used sparingly in the macrobiotic diet, so purchase them in small amounts. Most of them are high in fat and highly processed, and many use casein. Check the ingredients list on each product to make sure it doesn't contain milk proteins, look for organic brands, and experiment with several varieties to see which melt best and are the most palatable to you. Low-fat and fat-free varieties are available and are quite suitable for the recipes included in this book. If you're a cheese fan making the transition, you'll likely find the taste and texture of fat-free soy and rice cheeses bland and rubbery—stick to the regular varieties instead.

Fish

In the macrobiotic diet, fish is eaten in small quantities a few times a week. In macrobiotic terms, slow-moving, white-meat fish and shellfish, such as flounder, sole, cod, whitefish, clams, oysters, scallops, mussels, and octopus, are more yin and are considered preferable to fast-moving, dark-meat, more yang fish like tuna, salmon, herring, eel, trout, shrimp, lobster, crab, and squid. Since fish is eaten only a few times a week at most, buy it just before cooking—schedule a stop at the store on your way home from work. Purchase your fish from a reputable retailer, and remember that in general, the larger the store, the greater the turnover—and, therefore, the fresher the fish. In many cases, large chain stores will have the freshest fish, since they have the fastest turnover.

Look for firm flesh with little or no fishy smell. If you're buying fish whole, check the eyeballs—they should be clear, bright, and shiny, with no film. The skin should have a firm texture and should be slightly slimy and moist, again with little or no fish smell. Fattier fish—such as salmon and tuna—aren't as safe to eat, since toxins are stored in fat tissue. Stick to white-meat fish and shellfish. Farm-raised fish are an option as well. They're raised in a controlled environment and are generally exposed to less pollution and toxins.

Beans and Legumes

As a readily available source of high-quality, low-fat protein, beans are a standard in macrobiotic cooking. They can be served in countless incarnations, adding flavor, color, and texture to soups, casseroles, and stews; they can be made into salads with sea vegetables and grains, or they can round out a meal as a side dish. Many varieties of beans may also be sprouted and served as salads or garnishes. The most frequently used varieties of beans include azuki (aduki) beans, black-eyed peas, garbanzos (chickpeas), kidney beans, lentils, mung beans, green peas or split peas, and soybeans. Most beans can be bought in bulk at natural-products stores. Purchase the organic variety whenever possible, and always buy them whole and dried, never canned or frozen. Beans have a relatively long shelf life and do not need to be purchased on a weekly basis. Store them in a cool, dark place in tightly sealed containers.

GRAINS AND NOODLES

A variety of grains and noodles is essential in the macrobiotic kitchen. Buy them in bulk for the greatest savings and store them, labeled, in airtight glass containers in your cupboards. A colorful array of grains and noodles in decorative, clear-glass containers is an aesthetically pleasing addition to kitchen counters or exposed shelves. Just keep them out of direct sunlight and make sure they're well sealed.

Grains

Whole brown rice is, of course, the well-known mainstay of the macrobiotic diet, but many other varieties of rice and grains are staples to have on hand for soups, salads, casseroles and side dishes. The most commonly used rices include the following:

- Long-grain brown rice, the staple grain, with a nutty flavor and light, fluffy texture
- Medium-grain brown rice, slightly smaller and less elongated, with a softer, more moist texture than long-grain brown rice
- Short-grain brown rice, the smallest grain, with the most minerals and a high concentration of gluten
- Sweet brown rice, a faster cooking rice with a sweet taste and sticky texture and a high protein concentration
- Basmati, an aromatic and flavorful rice grown primarily in India and Thailand (also called popcorn rice for its distinctive aroma)
- Kokuko rose rice, a short-grain, sticky rice with a gelatinous texture (also called sushi rice)
- Wild rice, a grass seed with a strong flavor, usually combined with other types of rices

Stock your kitchen with a variety of other grains, including barley, buckwheat, corn (flour, grits, and meal), millet, oats, and wheat (germ, flour, and bulghur). Most grains and rice can be purchased in bulk at natural-products stores. Buy the organic variety whenever possible, and store them in tightly sealed glass containers in a cool, dark cupboard or in decorative containers out of direct sunlight.

Noodles

Noodles have a long and varied history in the Japanese and macrobiotic diets. Soba noodles (*soba* means "buckwheat" and also translates to "close by") were first introduced around 710 in Japan, not as the long, cylindrical shape we recognize now but as a flat, round, tortillalike concoction of buckwheat and water. They were eaten after being roasted over a fire.

The traditional preparation of noodles was a long and involved process wherein buckwheat flour dough was placed under straw tatami mats and kneaded thoroughly by stepping on the mats. After the dough became soft, it was rolled out on large wood cutting tables, pressed into a thin layer, and cut into narrow strips; it was then placed in a large kettle over a wood fire. After the noodles were cooked, cold mountain spring water was added to the kettle to halt the boiling, and after they had cooled, they were brought to a boil again. This process was repeated three or four times; the noodles were then removed and cooled, washed, and stacked for storage in bamboo boxes.

Noodles as we know them did not appear until the 1700s. At first, soba noodles were served in one of three forms: mori (noodles served separately with a sauce on the side), kake (noodles served in soup), and soba-gaki (a dish made of buckwheat flour mixed with hot water and eaten with sauce). New dishes soon evolved, some of which include

- Tempura soba (vegetable or shrimp tempura served over noodles in a soup base)
- Yamakake soba (noodles topped with grated radish or potato and served as a soup)
- Tsukimi soba (egg dropped on top of a bowl of noodles in a soup base)
- Ankakae soba (noodles topped with kuzu sauce and served as a soup)
- Mori soba (noodles topped with grated daikon radish, soy sauce, scallions, and nori)
- Kaki tama soba (a soup made of small pieces of deep-fried batter left over from tempura cooking)
- Kitsune soba (noodles topped with age, which is fried tofu)

Noodles are a fast-cooking, convenient way to add grains to your diet. The mainstays in the traditional macrobiotic diet include soba noodles and udon noodles. Soba noodles are made with buckwheat flour, probably the most yang grain. For this reason, they're generally served in colder climates. Several varieties of soba noodles (generally made with about 80 percent buckwheat flour and 20 percent wheat flour to facilitate the formation of the noodles) are available, including ftho soba, a short, thin variety; jenenjo soba, which contains mountain potato flour; cha soba, made with tea leaves and buckwheat; and youmugi soba, made with buckwheat and mugwort. Udon noodles are made from wheat. They are more yin in nature and were traditionally eaten in southern Japan, where the climate is warmer. Fresh udon noodles are thick and soft, while the dried variety is considerably thinner. Udon is traditionally made from sifted, or refined, flour, but it's also available made with 80–100 percent whole-wheat flour.

Ramen noodles (available fresh or dried) are a traditional Chinese noodle and are precooked by deep-fat frying—keep this in mind when you're calculating your fat intake. Somen noodles—thin, light noodles generally served cold in summer dishes—and saifun or cellophane noodles made from mung beans are also used in macrobiotic cooking. Various other whole-grain noodles—from corn elbow macaroni to whole-wheat spaghetti—add variety and interest. Dried noodles can be purchased in bulk and have a relatively long shelf life. Store them in a cool, dry cupboard.

NUTS AND SEEDS

Nuts and seeds are used in small quantities in macrobiotic cooking—as are nut and seed butters—as snacks, garnishes, and seasonings and to add flavor and texture to grain and vegetable salads and dishes. The nuts and seeds most frequently used in the macrobiotic diet are those that are dense and compact. Large, oily nuts and nuts from tropical climates are generally avoided. The most frequently used nuts include almonds, pine nuts, walnuts, chestnuts, and pecans; staple seeds include sesame seeds, sunflower seeds, and pumpkin seeds or pepitas.

The oils in nuts and seeds turn rancid quickly, so buy them in small quantities and use them within a week. Unshelled nuts are generally of the highest quality and have a longer shelf life than the shelled or hulled varieties, but they are obviously less convenient to use. Buy whole nuts rather than chopped, sliced, or slivered ones, since the whole varieties retain vital nutrients and food energy. Store nuts and seeds in a cool, dark cupboard or, if you can't use them within a week, keep them refrigerated to prevent spoilage and rancidity.

Nut and seed butters are also used for seasonings in soups, as dessert toppings, and for dressings and sauces. Tahini, made from ground sesame seeds, is the most frequently used butter. Sunflower butter and almond butter are also used in many of the recipes in this book, and peanut butter and cashew butter may be used in very small quantities in dressings and sauces. Avoid the processed nut and seed butters found in supermarkets, especially peanut butter—they generally contain preservatives and sweeteners. Many nut and seed butters are available in bulk at natural-products stores—they're less expensive and can be purchased in small quantities. Buy the organic varieties whenever possible, and buy them in small quantities, since ground nuts and seeds lose their nutritional value and food energy quickly and are more susceptible to spoilage and rancidity. Store nuts and seed butters in a cool, dark cupboard after opening, and try to use them within one week.

THE BASIC UTENSILS

While the methods and recipes described in this book will not necessitate that you rewire your kitchen or spend a month's wages on cooking apparatus at your local specialty store, some specific utensils are helpful and often necessary for macrobiotic cooking. Wherever possible, the American versions of these utensils are listed.

A gas stove is always preferable to an electric stove. According to the macrobiotic philosophy, the yang energy imparted to foods through gas is more balanced than the energy from electric heat, and, in terms of practicality and manageability, gas stoves are infinitely superior—something to keep in mind if you're remodeling or moving in the near future. Otherwise, an electric range will suffice.

You'll be able to get by with an electric blender (the hand-held types are by far more versatile), the standard selection of pots and pans, some wooden spoons, and a few specialty items that can be found in most natural-products stores or Oriental markets (these items are discussed below). If your kitchen is cramped for space, you'll find that most specialty utensils are infinitely more attractive than the standard American cooking gear and can be hung by nails on the walls of your kitchen, where they're more easily accessible. Many of these items are made of bamboo and must be air-dried to prevent mildewing, so hanging is also a practical way to store them. Suribachis and other pottery items can be stowed in the corners of your kitchen counters as exotic, decorative touches.

Saucepans should have tight-fitting lids and heavy bottoms to conduct heat more evenly. They should be made of stainless steel, cast iron, glass, or enamel. Aluminum and Teflon pans are generally not recommended. Cast-iron skillets are versatile and well worth the investment, since they heat slowly and distribute heat more uniformly. Cast-iron cookware should be seasoned by first coating the inside with sesame oil, then heating it in a 250°F oven for a couple of hours and allowing it to cool overnight. Clean cast iron by washing in hot water and drying over a low flame to prevent rusting. If food sticks to the bottom, use a little coarse sea salt to scrub it off, then rinse with hot water. Flame deflectors are used under saucepans and pressure cookers to distribute heat evenly during cooking and to prevent burning. They are essential if you're cooking with pottery.

Wooden spoons, wooden rice paddles, and other utensils made from wood are the most durable and desirable for stirring and serving, since they impart no taste to the food, won't chip enamel pots, and don't tear delicate vegetables and noodles while stirring. Long-handled chopsticks, called *hashi,* are also used for stirring in deep pots and for frying.

Cutting boards should be made of wood rather than plastic, which is slippery and allows knives to slip easily. To clean wooden boards, rub salt into the surface, rinse in cold water, dry well, and coat lightly with sesame oil.

An assortment of glass jars is necessary for storing grains, legumes, and seasonings. If you're storing salt-based seasonings, such as gomashio, make sure the glass container doesn't have a rubber ring around the top—the salt will corrode it and loosen the seal.

Specialty Items

The suribachi, a deep ceramic bowl, has narrow grooves and sloping sides. It is used with a wooden pestle (*surikogi*) to grind sesame seeds for gomashio, to powder sea vegetables for seasonings, and to mix miso, dressings, dips, and sauces. The medium-size suribachi (about ten inches in diameter) is the most versatile; however, a good-size mortar and pestle works just as well.

Sushi mats (*maki-su*) are used to make nori rolls and as covers for serving bowls to retain heat while allowing steam to escape. They are also used to cover leftovers, letting them breathe without drying out.

Strainers are used to drain vegetables and noodles after cooking, to rinse and toss salads, and to strain twig teas. Bamboo baskets (*zaru*) are the traditional forms of strainers, but colanders may also be used.

A stainless-steel steamer may be used for most vegetables, but bamboo steamers (*mushiki*) are preferable, since the bamboo won't alter the taste of the food during cooking. Most *mushiki* come in sets of two or three tiers, which are filled with separate foods, covered with a lid, and placed over a pot of boiling water.

Known as *tawashi,* natural coconut-fiber brushes are the best choices for scrubbing vegetables. The bristles are soft enough to scrub delicate-skinned vegetables without damaging the surfaces, yet they are firm enough to clean root vegetables well, eliminating the need to peel them.

Grain and spice mills are used to grind fresh seeds and nuts for butters and spreads, to grind whole grains into flours, and to process whole spices, like cumin seed and peppers, for seasonings. Freshly ground nut butters and flours are far superior to commercially ground products in terms of flavor and nutritional value. Coffee grinders are sufficient for most purposes. If you grind your own coffee beans, however, purchase a second grinder or mill for spices and nut butters, unless you particularly enjoy the taste of tahini or cumin in your morning coffee.

Stainless-steel graters are needed for carrots and other root vegetables, and porcelain or ceramic graters (*oroshigane*) are ideal for grating spicy roots such as ginger and radish. Traditional macrobiotic cooking uses graters that grate foods more finely than commercial graters.

Casserole dishes are used for baking root vegetables and grain dishes. The traditional Japanese casserole (*donabe*) is a thick-walled dish made of earthenware and can be used on top of the stove as well as in the oven. It retains heat well and distributes it evenly during the cooking process. Glass casseroles in several sizes may also be used.

Pressure cookers are a standard in most macrobiotic kitchens. They cook grains and legumes much more quickly and reliably than other methods, and they help retain more vitamins and other nutrients. Stainless-steel pressure cookers are preferable to aluminum.

A wok is especially useful for stir-frying and preparing tempura dishes. The sloping sides of the wok allow for a larger surface area and more uniform cooking. Several varieties are available, from the traditional cast-iron version with a rounded bottom which sits on a small, circular stand, to the flat-bottomed version that is more practical for electric ranges.

5

COOKING TECHNIQUES
AND TRADITIONS

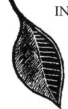

IN ADDITION TO DIETARY COMPONENTS, there are other more subtle ways in which macrobiotic practices promote optimal health in the Western diet. A certain, pervasive social order in eating exists in Japanese and Oriental traditions. Food preparation is careful and meticulous, cooking helps maintain the balance of yin and yang, and presentation and ritual are significant parts of the Oriental way of eating. George Ohsawa advised eating with other people as often as possible as a way to share the life energy of foods and to make it more likely that you will eat moderately and sensibly.

The Western tradition of cooking and food preparation has an almost singular focus on the physical content of the diet. In the Oriental tradition, foods are prepared with great care and concentration and with a positive attitude, which is thought to impart healthful value and a subtle, intangible energy to the food. The Eastern tradition believes that one receives from the meal what he or she has put into it. Food that is prepared with a calm, attentive mind and attitude, rather than thrown together in a frenzied, stressful rush, has the ability to nourish the body, mind, and spirit. A meal prepared with love, care, and tranquility will impart a high quantity and quality of life-giving nutrients as well as intangible energy, or what the Japanese call Ki. The idea of eating is to nourish body, mind, and spirit; or, in Western terms, eat to live, don't live to eat.

General Preparation Techniques for Vegetables

The method and manner in which foods are cut and prepared for cooking is of utmost importance in macrobiotic cooking. Wash and scrub root and ground vegetables gently, being careful not to damage the skin. Completely immerse leafy greens in fresh water and soak briefly to remove dirt or sand; then drain thoroughly. A salad spinner is helpful, if you have one, or use a bamboo basket or colander. Completely immerse mushrooms in water and soak briefly, then drain them thoroughly and gently pat dry before slicing.

A Note on Knives and Cutting Techniques

Macrobiotic philosophy places a great deal of attention and emphasis on cutting techniques, for both aesthetic and nutritional reasons. A variety of shapes and sizes lends considerable visual appeal to any dish, and the ways in which vegetables are cut are important in maintaining the highest level of yin/yang balance.

If you've been hacking away at carrots with the same rusty paring knife you received as a wedding present or the meat cleaver your grandmother gave you for college graduation, spend a few dollars on well-made knives and a sharpener. High-quality sushi knives are available in Oriental markets and at most department stores, and a knife sharpener is a worthwhile investment as well. Whatever knives you choose to use, make sure they're sharp and don't have nicks or rusty edges.

Traditional macrobiotic cooking and preparation involves some initially tricky maneuvers with knives. The following methods of cutting can be used as you wish—interpret them as liberally as is practical for your needs. Generally, however, roots are sliced diagonally, and round or aboveground vegetables are cut from top to bottom to expose an equal quantity of yin and yang properties in each portion.

Hangetsu Giri

HANGETSU GIRI

For thick, cylindrical vegetables, such as cucumbers and turnips, use the *hangetsu giri* method of cutting. The vegetable is sliced in half lengthwise, then cut into half moons.

HASU GIRI

The most common form of cutting vegetables in Japanese and macrobiotic cooking is *hasu giri*. This technique is especially useful for root vegetables such as carrots and daikon. The idea is to provide as much yin and yang in each cut portion of the vegetable as possible by exposing both the outside and the inside. Vegetables are cut on an angle into thin, diagonal slices.

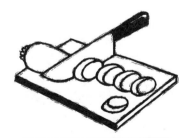

Hasu Giri

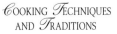

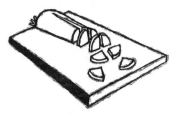

Icho Giri

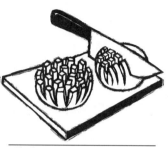

Kikuka Giri

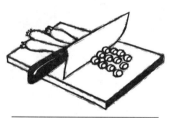

Koguchi Giri

Mawashi Giri

ICHO GIRI

Icho giri is used most often for long, thick vegetables such as squash and sweet potatoes. Cut the vegetables in half lengthwise; then cut each half lengthwise again, yielding four long quarters. Line the quarters up and slice crosswise to create heart-shaped quarter moons.

KIKUKA GIRI

Kikuka giri is a decorative cutting technique used mostly for garnishes with round root vegetables or aboveground vegetables. Slice off the very top of the vegetable to create a flat surface, then place the vegetable between a pair of chopsticks to steady it during cutting. Make a series of thin, lengthwise cuts across the top of the vegetable, stopping about $1/2$ inch short of the bottom. Turn the vegetable and cut in the opposite direction, the same thickness. Soak the vegetable in ice water for half an hour to allow it to "bloom" into a flower shape.

KOGUCHI GIRI

Used mostly for scallions and other long, thin vegetables, the *koguchi giri* method involves cutting thin, round slices straight across the vegetable.

MAWASHI GIRI

The *mawashi giri* technique is used mainly on round vegetables, especially onions. In Japanese, the word *mawashi* translates into "turn." Cut the vegetable in half vertically, then cut thin vertical slices, holding the vegetable upright and rotating it as you cut.

MIJIN GIRI

Similar to mincing, *mijin giri* can be used on most vegetables and is especially suited to onions and ginger. Cut the vegetable in half, then hold each half cut-side down and cut horizontally (as in the *sainome* style) in very thin slices, then diagonally, again in very thin slices.

RAN GIRI

The unique *ran giri* method of cutting vegetables is ideal for soups and stews and lends an interesting look to stir-fries. *Ran giri* can be used on most root vegetables, especially elongated ones. Cut thick vegetables in half first; make a diagonal cut across the vegetable, then turn it 180 degrees and make a similar cut in the same direction, creating irregular chunks with diagonal surface areas.

SAINOME

Similar to the technique of cubing, *sainome* is best suited to larger vegetables. Cut the vegetable in half lengthwise, then place each half cut-side down on the board. Slice horizontally in even thicknesses, then, keeping the horizontal slices together, cut vertically to create cubes. The size of the cubes depends on the cooking techniques to be used: The cubes will be larger for soups, stews, and casseroles than for stir-fries.

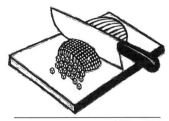

Mijin Giri

SASAGAKI

Used mainly for burdock root, *sasagaki* is similar to sharpening a pencil with a knife. Hold the burdock root at the top end and lightly shave the root in a downward stroke, using a very sharp knife and turning the burdock as you shave it. *Sasagaki* may also be used for carrots and other long, slender vegetables.

SEN GIRI

Similar to the technique of julienne or matchstick cutting styles, *sen giri* is best suited to long, thick root vegetables. Cut the vegetable on the diagonal in the *hasu giri* style, then cut each diagonal piece into thin matchsticks. This method is best suited to quick-cooking dishes and for salads.

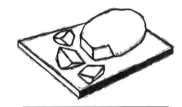

Ran Giri

TANZAKU

The unique cutting style of the *tanzaku* method yields rectangular slices of vegetables and adds aesthetic value to stir-fries and steamed dishes. *Tanzaku* is used most often on long root vegetables and some larger aboveground vegetables. Cut the vegetable horizontally into one- to two-inch sections; slice each section vertically into about three slices, and then cut each slice lengthwise into thinner slices to make long, rectangular pieces.

WA GIRI

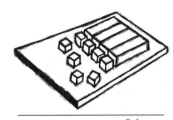

Sainome

The *wa giri* technique is similar to *koguchi giri*, which involves cutting thin, round slices straight across the vegetable, but it is generally used for thick vegetables such as carrots. *Wa giri* yields thicker slices than the *koguchi giri* style.

MACRO COOKING TECHNIQUES

Traditional macrobiotic cooking uses a variety of cooking methods, all of which are designed to maintain the balance of yin and yang in the dishes, to render the foods most palatable, and to preserve the highest nutritional value possible. Some popular theories hold that raw foods are among the most nutritionally acceptable foods and that cooking destroys vitamins and other nutrients. Not necessarily true—or, rather, it all depends. Long cooking times over high heat will, indeed, destroy most valuable enzymes and some vitamins in foods, but macrobiotic methods of cooking and preparation are designed to maintain the nutritional value of foods.

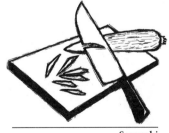

Sasagaki

Cooking is the first step in digestion. It helps break down cellulose walls

Sen Giri

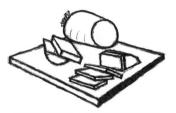

Tanzaku

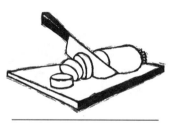

Wa Giri

in vegetables, thereby rendering the nutrients more bioavailable and making them easier for the body to assimilate. Raw broccoli may have a minutely higher level of enzymes and slightly more vitamins than lightly steamed broccoli, but if those nutrients are unavailable to your body, you've essentially wasted the food you're eating. Which is not to say that raw food is to be excluded from the diet entirely. Sprouted and other raw, "living" foods contain valuable enzymes that are nutritionally viable and essential for overall health. But, in general, cooked foods are more bioavailable to the body and offer the most balanced blend of nutrients and yin/yang qualities.

Four elements, or forces, in food preparation are recognized in traditional macrobiotic cooking: fire, salt, pressure, and time. Cooking methods that use fire or heat include boiling, steaming, sautéing, baking, broiling, deep-frying, and pressure-cooking, all of which will be discussed in greater detail shortly.

Fire, a highly yang influence, neutralizes the acid content of yin foods, thereby allowing the yang energy to be extracted and permitting the food to become more balanced. For example, corn is considered relatively yin, and cooking balances that yin energy with yang influences. Thus, cooked corn has a more balanced yin/yang energy than raw corn.

Salting as a "cooking" or pickling method uses pure, unrefined sea salt, which is rich in trace minerals, including magnesium, calcium, phosphorus, iron, and iodine. Miso, tamari, and umeboshi are also used for "cooking" or pickling vegetables and other foods for condiments.

Pressure and time are two additional methods of "cooking" used in the macrobiotic diet. Pickles and pressed salads are the most common dishes that use these techniques. Pressure is a yin force, and the combination of time, pressure, and salt used to prepare, for example, pickled vegetables neutralizes excess acid in the foods and helps break down tough cellulose walls that make nutrients unavailable. Pressure-cooking—traditionally used for rice—is another way in which pressure is used.

In general, leafy greens and most aboveground vegetables, such as squash, broccoli, and cauliflower, require short cooking times. They may be steamed lightly in a bamboo or stainless-steel steamer or cooked in an inch or two of water. More delicate leafy greens, like lettuces and baby spinach, can be barely wilted by dropping them into about 1/2 inch of boiling water or by steaming them for about thirty seconds. Root vegetables require longer cooking times and are better suited for boiling or cooking in a small amount of oil. Tofu, tempeh, and other bean products should be cooked thoroughly to aid digestion, and legumes and grains require more specialized cooking techniques, which will be discussed shortly.

Boiling

Contrary to popular belief, boiling vegetables does not cause substantial nutrient loss if done properly. Boiling is a more yin method of cooking and is best suited to root vegetables and heavier aboveground vegetables. Use only a small amount of water—about one to two inches at most—with a pinch of unrefined sea salt; bring the water to a full boil before adding vegetables to seal in nutrients and color. Simmer on low heat until just tender. Serve boiled vegetables immediately to prevent loss of color and nutritional value (and save the water to use for soup stocks).

Soups and stews are prepared by boiling, but they require more water to make a broth. For a simple, traditional macrobiotic soup, drop a variety of vegetables into boiling water. Add a strip of kombu and a pinch of unrefined sea salt. After about five minutes, add noodles, tofu, or tempeh and other sea vegetables. Cook for ten more minutes or until noodles are done and vegetables are tender. Remove kombu, and add miso, shoyu, gomashio, or other seasonings.

Boiling is also used to make traditional boiled salads. To make boiled salads, bring about ½ inch of water and a pinch of unrefined sea salt to a full boil. Use watercress, cabbage, Chinese cabbage, onions, carrots, kale, daikon, or almost any other vegetable. Drop the vegetables into the boiling water, adding those with the mildest flavors first and removing each before adding the next type of vegetable. Cook for one or two minutes, or until just wilted (boil carrots and daikon for about two minutes or until brightly colored and still crispy). Drain and rinse immediately with cold water to stop cooking, and combine vegetables or serve separately in small dishes.

Steaming

Steaming, one of the best methods for cooking leafy green vegetables, retains the color and nutritional value of the vegetables. A variety of vegetables can be steamed together—start with the dense, hard vegetables first, then add softer vegetables and greens toward the end of cooking, after the harder vegetables are barely tender. Bring ½ inch of water and a pinch of unrefined sea salt to a full boil. Place vegetables in a stainless-steel or bamboo steamer; place the steamer in the pot, and cover with a tight-fitting lid, cooking just until tender and still crisp.

Sautéing

Most vegetables can be sautéed in a small amount of unrefined vegetable oil at medium temperatures (heating oils to extremely high temperatures can result in the loss of vitamin E and the formation of free radicals). Use only as much oil as needed to lightly coat the bottom of the cooking utensil—try brushing the surface of the pot or pan with oil, using a natural bristle brush from the hardware store. In general, about two teaspoons of oil should be used for a dish that will serve four people. A pinch of unrefined sea salt sprinkled over the vegetables brings out their natural sweetness and causes them to give up their juices, decreasing the need for oil. To sauté, heat a small amount of oil in a skillet or wok over medium heat, add the vegetables, and stir them gently with a wooden utensil until tender (about five minutes, depending on the cutting style and type of vegetable used). Turn the heat down and cover with a tight-fitting lid if you're sautéing root or dense aboveground vegetables, or cook uncovered if you're sautéing leafy greens or vegetables with a high water content. Sauté, stirring gently and occasionally to prevent sticking and burning, for five to ten more minutes, or until tender. A small amount of water or sake may also be added to prevent sticking.

Baking or Roasting

Almost any vegetable can be baked or roasted, but this method is best suited to root vegetables, winter squashes, and peppers and is most often used during colder seasons. Use a glass or cast-iron casserole dish, or purchase a *donabe,* an eminently versatile ceramic Japanese dish that can be used on top of the stove as well as in the oven. When baking vegetables, coat the bottom of the casserole lightly with oil to prevent sticking, and stir gently once or twice during the cooking process to ensure even cooking. Cook at 350°F to 375°F until tender. Tempeh and seitan can also be added to the vegetables for a convenient, one-dish meal. Season with shoyu or tamari and gomashio.

Broiling

A variety of vegetables can be broiled—onions, peppers, and mushrooms are especially delicious prepared this way. They should be lightly brushed with sesame oil to keep them from drying out (basting sauces may also be used). Fish, tofu, tempeh, and seitan are also well suited for broiling. To broil vegetables, fish, or bean products, toss ingredients in a basting sauce or brush them sparingly with sesame oil, and arrange them one layer deep in a glass casserole lightly coated with sesame oil. Place the casserole on the lowest rung in the oven, and stir occasionally to keep the ingredients from sticking and burning or drying out.

Deep Frying

Used mainly in winter months and in colder climates, deep-frying requires more oil than other methods and is therefore used less frequently. Done properly, however, deep-frying is a cooking technique that yields a warming energy and a variety of textures to macrobiotic meals. Serve with ginger and tamari sauces and side dishes of grated daikon and pickled ginger to help neutralize the oil. Tempeh is especially tasty deep-fried, and vegetables and

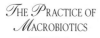

shellfish can be deep-fried tempura style by dipping them in a flour and water batter and dropping them into the hot oil. Light sesame oil (rather than dark, roasted sesame oil), safflower oil, and sunflower oil are best suited for deep-frying. Use about three inches of oil in a deep saucepan or wok, and heat oil to about 350°F to prevent food from becoming greasy and soggy. Temperatures higher than about 355°F will cause the ingredients to burn or cook on the outside while the inside remains raw. Drain vegetables and other ingredients on a rack or a platter covered with paper towels, and serve in a dish with a thick napkin to soak up any remaining oil.

SPECIAL COOKING TECHNIQUES FOR BEANS AND GRAINS

Beans and grains play such an important part in the macrobiotic diet that they warrant a little extra time and space to describe the specifics of preparing them, from selection and storage to cooking techniques.

Beans

Peas, beans, and peanuts, considered legumes, are rich in vitamins, minerals, and protein and may contain as much protein as animal products, or more. They're a rich source of calcium, iron, and B vitamins and, when sprouted, add valuable enzymes to the daily diet.

Because beans can be difficult to digest, there are some specific preparation and cooking techniques that should be followed to maximize nutritional value and digestibility. Buy beans in bulk at natural-products stores for the greatest savings and highest quality. Before cooking, sort them well, pick out small stones, and wash them thoroughly. Most beans must be soaked for a minimum of five hours—or, better yet, overnight. Lentils and split peas don't have to be soaked, since they cook quickly.

Place the beans in a large bowl or pot, cover them completely with hot water, and let them soak. Before cooking, discard the soaking water. Layer two five-inch-long strips of kombu on the bottom of a heavy-bottomed cooking pan to help the beans cook faster and to make them easier to digest. Rinse the beans again, and place one cup soaked beans and four cups fresh, cold water in the pan (don't add salt to the cooking water—it makes the beans tough). Bring the beans to a full boil, cover, and reduce heat to low, cooking until tender. The length of cooking time varies depending on the type of bean used (Table 7). Lentils can cook in forty minutes, while garbanzo beans need as long as four hours. When the beans are nearly done, add ¹/₂ teaspoon unrefined sea salt and cook until soft and thoroughly done.

Another method of cooking beans is called the shocking method. Again, place two strips of kombu on the bottom of a large, heavy pot. Add just enough water to cover the surface of the beans, bring to a full boil, and then reduce to a simmer. Use a pot cover that fits completely inside the cooking pot, and place it directly onto the beans to keep them stable and to reduce their cooking time. When the beans begin to expand, remove the lid and add just enough cold water to cover them, pouring the water carefully down the side of the pot. Replace the cover directly on top of the beans, and repeat the process until they're almost done. Remove the cover, add unrefined sea salt, and simmer until the beans are soft. Turn up the heat during the last few minutes to boil off excess water.

Table 7
COOKING TIMES FOR BEANS

BEAN	COOKING TIME (FOR SOAKED BEANS)
Azuki (aduki)	Boil 1½ hours. Pressure-cook about 7 minutes.
Anasazi	Boil 1 hour. Pressure-cook about 7 minutes.
Black turtle	Boil 1½–2 hours. Pressure-cook about 10 minutes.
Black-eyed peas	Boil 45 minutes. Pressure-cook about 10 minutes (soaking is not required).
Fava	Boil 3 hours. Pressure-cook about 15 minutes.
Garbanzos (chickpeas)	Boil 3–4 hours. Pressure-cook about 12–15 minutes.
Great Northern	Boil 1 hour. Pressure-cook about 10 minutes.
Kidney	Boil 1½ hours. Pressure-cook about 10 minutes.
Lentils	Boil 30–45 minutes. Pressure-cooking is not recommended (soaking is not required).
Lima	Boil 1½ to 2 hours. Pressure-cook about 7 minutes.
Mung	Boil 45 minutes to 1 hour. Pressure-cook about 10 minutes (soaking is not required).
Navy	Boil 2 hours. Pressure-cook about 10 minutes.
Peas (dried, split)	Boil 45 minutes. Pressure-cooking is not recommended (soaking is not required).
Pinto	Boil 1–1½ hours. Pressure-cook about 10 minutes.
Red	Boil 1½ hours. Pressure-cook about 15 minutes.
Soybean	Boil 3–4 hours. Pressure-cook about 45 minutes.

Grains

Rice and other grains are the mainstays of the macrobiotic diet, and a number of specific cooking techniques should be considered. There are essentially three types of brown rice: short grain, a sweet, sticky rice well suited to sushi and rice balls; medium grain, a moist, fluffy rice suitable for porridges and breakfast cereals, casseroles, and stuffings; and long grain, a very fluffy, light rice ideal for stir-fries.

In macrobiotic cooking, rice is generally prepared in a pressure cooker, a variation of the traditional Japanese method of preparation in which rice was cooked in a cast-iron pot with a heavy wooden lid. Pressure-cooking yields rice that's more uniformly cooked, slightly sweeter, and easier to digest. A pressure cooker is by no means a necessity, but it can be a valuable, time-saving addition to your kitchen.

If you're not ready to go the pressure-cooker route, rice and other grains can be prepared in a regular pot with a tight-fitting lid. Some grains may be soaked overnight to soften them and shorten the cooking time, and most grains may be toasted in the pot (before adding water) to enhance the flavor and impart a slightly nutty taste and aroma. In general, rinse grains just before cooking; use about one part grain to two to three parts water; add a pinch of unrefined sea salt; boil vigorously for five minutes, then lower the heat and cover with a tight-fitting lid; cook until water is absorbed (Table 8).

If you choose to use a pressure cooker, first place the rice in a bowl of cold water to wash it off, stirring it quickly with your hand and draining off the water in a colander. To make rice softer and more digestible, place it in a pressure cooker (one part rice to two parts water), cover it tightly, and soak for several hours or overnight. Add a pinch of unrefined sea salt, seal the pressure cooker, and cook for about twenty minutes.

If you don't have the time or inclination to soak the rice, toast it first for a nutty flavor, being careful not to burn or brown it. When the rice begins to become aromatic, add two parts water to one part rice and a pinch of sea salt; seal the pressure cooker and cook for about twenty minutes. Remove the rice from the pressure cooker as soon as it's finished cooking to prevent the moisture from making the rice gummy and wet. Use a damp rice paddle or wooden spoon, and serve a balanced blend of rice from the bottom and top of the pressure cooker.

The way in which rice is cooked in traditional macrobiotic cooking greatly influences its balance of yin and yang characteristics. To lend the rice a stronger yin, or cooling, influence, the rice is cooked on a low flame, which allows the pressure to build gradually, permitting the grains to adapt to the heat and yielding a sweet flavor. For a more yang, or warming, influence, rice is cooked over a high flame, which allows the pressure to build quickly before the heat is reduced, and the rice finishes cooking at a lower temperature.

Other grains can be prepared in pressure cookers as well, again with the same results—a sweeter, lighter grain that is more uniformly cooked and quickly prepared. Try cooking barley, wheat berries, millet, and various other grains, either alone or with rice, in a pressure cooker. Experiment by adding wild rice, red rice, and other varieties of rice. The possibilities are nearly endless.

Table 8
COOKING GRAINS

GRAIN	AMOUNT OF WATER (FOR 1 CUP GRAIN)	COOKING TIME
Barley	3 cups	1½ hours
Brown rice	2 cups	30–40 minutes
Buckwheat	2 cups	20–30 minutes
Bulghur	2 cups	15–20 minutes
Couscous	1½ cups	15 minutes
Millet	2½ cups	20 minutes
Oats	2½ cups	20–30 minutes
Polenta	3 cups	20 minutes
Quinoa	2 cups	15–20 minutes
Wild rice	4 cups	45 minutes to 1 hour

PRESENTATION AND PRODUCTION

In our modern world of cooking and cuisine, food preparation may end the minute the pots are plucked from the burners. We may spend considerable time at the grocery store, select the best produce and the freshest fish, carefully chop and cut vegetables, combine and cook all ingredients with the utmost awareness and attention to detail. But once the dish is done, we lose all sense of attention, awareness, and aesthetic appeal. An appointed family member sets the table in a frenzied rush, dropping the nearest utensils at hand onto place mats that may or may not match. Food is plopped onto the plates, the chef of the night bellows "Dinner!" and the family gathers for the meal, paying little attention to table settings, production, and presentation. The food is on the plate. What more do we need?

Much more, according to the principles of macrobiotics. The presentation of a meal is crucial in the macrobiotic diet, which is not to say that the table must be appointed with crystal goblets, sterling silver cutlery, and china plates. Rather, the table should be set in a way that continues and furthers the aesthetic appeal of the meal. Fresh flowers, matching plates and place mats, cloth napkins, and the proper eating and serving utensils go a long way toward making any meal memorable.

This macrobiotic maxim doesn't apply only to family dinners. Even brown-bag lunches eaten at your desk at work can be visually appealing and aesthetically pleasing and should receive the highest degree of attention to presentation. If you tote your lunch to work in a crumpled brown bag with plastic forks and paper towels, then toss it in the microwave and gulp it down during meetings or monthly budget reviews, you're missing a great deal of the macrobiotic concept of eating and balance.

Make your lunches as important as every other meal of the day. Take glass or ceramic dishes on which to serve your food, chopsticks or flatware, and a cloth napkin. Set aside at least half an hour, eating slowly and thoughtfully and chewing well. If possible, try to eat somewhere other than your desk, and take a ten- or fifteen-minute walk outside once your meal is finished.

When serving food at any meal, maintain a sense of balance and proportion. Arrange food carefully on the plates, being aware of colors and textures and how they mix and blend. Don't heap dishes with mounds of food—you can always go back for seconds. As the macrobiotic maxim says, "From one grain, ten thousand grains." That is, if everyone in the world threw away one grain of rice, millions of grains—which could feed thousands of people or grow enough to feed millions more—would be lost.

One-dish meals, such as stews and casseroles, can be presented in earthenware, glass, or pottery serving dishes and then brought to the table in the traditional Oriental family-style manner of serving. If you have a number of side dishes, try presenting them in smaller bowls to be passed around the table. And don't limit your imagination when it comes to presentation. Bowls and platters aren't the only alternatives to serving dishes. Try serving foods in hollowed-out zucchini and pumpkin shells or on leaves and steamed greens that can become part of the meal.

Garnish plates with edible flowers or sprigs of fresh herbs such as parsley, cilantro, basil, or marjoram. Sprinkle grain or noodle dishes with gomashio, poppy seeds, nuts, or a small amount of coarsely ground black pepper. Use vegetable garnishes such as radish roses, cucumber crescents, thinly sliced scallions, and pickled ginger or daikon root for color and added interest. Also include small dishes of condiments and pickles for balance, digestion, and aesthetic appeal. Before beginning to eat, breathe deeply and observe the array of food before you, giving thanks for the meal in whatever manner you may choose.

PART THREE

Making Macrobiotics Work for You

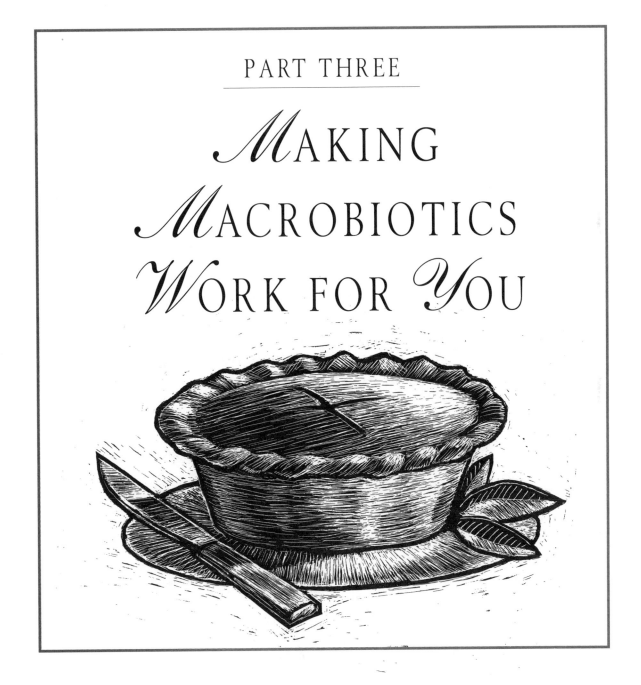

6

"FORBIDDEN" FOODS
The Traditional Approach

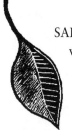 SAINTS THESE DAYS ARE FEW and far between, and most of us would find life without the occasional mango (or glass of wine or shot of espresso) scarcely worth living. It's possible to have your cake (or mangos or wine or espresso) every once in a while and still live quite well. Macrobiotics is about choice, and if you choose to "cheat" on the macro mandates, it's your prerogative.

One point should be perfectly clear: Some foods are so extreme in their makeup that including them on a daily basis or in excessive quantities will wreak constant havoc and irreparable damage on your body, mind, and spirit. Specific foods are forbidden in the strict macrobiotic diet, which was originally a healing regimen—a program designed to cure illness. Unless you're sick, however, there's nothing wrong with breaking the rules every once in a while. Excessive guilt and self-flagellation are unquestionably more detrimental to your overall health than an occasional avocado. Even George Ohsawa, in his *Macrobiotic Guide Book for Living,* says "I enjoy any cuisine. . . . I like fruit, candy, chocolate and whiskey very much. If I choose to use these things now I am able to avoid harm because I can balance yin and yang. We must choose what is good for us—the art of making such a choice is macrobiotics." So let's talk about the forbidden foods, why the macrobiotic diet eschews them, and why it's probably permissible to eat them occasionally, with awareness of their detrimental health effects.

This somewhat controversial chapter was composed with a small measure of wariness, so I feel compelled to make a disclaimer of sorts. First, even though the founder of any movement may bend or break the rules at times, that doesn't give the rest of us carte blanche to run roughshod over the principles of the practice. The preceding quote from Ohsawa was included to illustrate that even the most rigid of practitioners recognizes that personal choices for occasional indulgences, with a sense of awareness, are permissible. The operative terms to keep in mind while reading this chapter are *occasional* and *awareness*. This book is not meant to chastise or proselytize; it was written as a sincere attempt to dispense ethical advice and maintain nutritional integrity. Remember that *occasional* means once or twice a week and that *awareness* means making clear and conscious personal decisions armed with knowledge, information, and the understanding that the foods you are about to eat may be hazardous to your health. Or, to repeat the words of Ohsawa, "We must choose what is good for us—the art of making such a choice is macrobiotics."

The Macro No-Nos: Never Say "Never"

White Sugar

The topic of refined white sugar has been discussed at length in preceding chapters, and it's been established that high sugar consumption is undeniably detrimental. Excessive sugar consumption has been linked to tooth decay, hyperactivity, high blood pressure, diabetes, obesity, stress on the pancreas and adrenals, manic behavior, schizophrenia, and numerous other mental disorders. Refined white sugar also depletes nutrients in the body, reduces digestive enzymes and hydrochloric acid, and causes sharp fluctuations in blood sugar levels.

Given all of the above, remember that if you're in overall good health, an occasional chocolate chip cookie probably won't render you incapable of functioning. We're all continually confronted with countless opportunities to cheat, so choose your poisons carefully. Be aware of the foods you eat that contain sugar, and watch out for its insidious inclusion in hidden sources. Many refined foods, including breakfast cereals, breads, and crackers, contain as much as 50 percent sugar, and refined sweeteners in the guise of high-fructose corn syrup, sucrose, and dextrose crop up regularly in the most unexpected foods and condiments.

If you decide to "cheat," do it with dignity and limit yourself to a few bites of the culprit. Slowly savor every morsel, rather than mindlessly chomping away. In other words, if you decide to break the rules once in a while, do it with acute awareness, and remember that it's not really the white sugar that's acceptable, it's the "once in a while" that's okay.

Coffee

Countless alternatives to coffee are recommended in the macrobiotic diet, but if you're accustomed to a rich mug of cappuccino for your morning motivation, roasted grain beverages may seem like pale imitations and will hardly satisfy a discerning palate.

Coffee is the equivalent of a poison, if you subscribe to the speculations of most health practitioners and nutritionists. Coffee is a psychologically and physically addictive drug. It's heavily treated with systemic chemical fertilizers and pesticides; the roasting process used to prepare coffee may cause the beans to become mutagenic; and the caffeine content in coffee is detrimental to kidney function and the nervous system.

Nor is decaffeinated coffee the panacea it's purported to be. The most widely used method of decaffeinating coffee involves the use of solvents, generally methylene chloride, which leaves solvent residues in the coffee. Two other methods of decaffeination are available. The first, water processing, retains most of the volatile oils and, therefore, flavor of the coffee, and eliminates more caffeine. A second but less widely used method is the carbon-dioxide processing method, which uses no harmful chemicals and retains the highest amount of flavor.

There are two basic types of coffee bean: robusta and arabica. Robusta blends have a cruder, more bitter flavor and aroma than arabica blends and are higher in caffeine (190 milligrams per six-ounce cup compared with 140 milligrams). These are the types of coffee generally served in truck stops, convenience stores, and cheap restaurants. Arabica blends are to coffee what varietal grapes are to wines. These varieties are found in most specialty shops and gourmet purveyors and have markedly different flavors and aromas than robusta blends.

While coffee is one of the most heavily sprayed food crops in the world, coffee beans don't contain an inordinately high concentration of pesticides, since the beans themselves are contained in small, fruitlike berries. There is some systemic integration of pesticides into the beans, yet so many organic coffees are now available that pesticide residue should be small cause for concern. Organic coffees come primarily from Central America, and some Indonesian and Hawaiian Island coffees are now available in certified organic blends.

Espresso—even though it's rich and flavorful and has a stronger taste than regular brewed coffee—imparts less caffeine: A shot of espresso delivers about sixty to ninety milligrams of caffeine. Espresso uses a finer grind with a smaller surface area. During the brewing process, steaming hot water is forced through the coffee for eighteen to twenty-three seconds, versus the three to five minutes required for drip or brewed coffee. The end result is that the water is in contact with the coffee for a much shorter time, thereby leaching considerably less caffeine from the coffee grinds into your cup.

This is not meant to advocate the uninhibited imbibing of coffee. If you do drink coffee, limit your consumption to an infrequent amount—one six- to eight-ounce cup two or three times a week—and stick to organically grown coffees and brewing methods that yield more flavor and a lower caffeine content. With the abundance of specialty shops and organic coffee blends on the market, no reason exists for you to slurp down pesticide-laden, traditionally brewed commercial coffees.

While there's no hard evidence that you need to eschew coffee completely and forever, if you feel you must have a cup every single morning to function normally, you might want to reexamine your thinking about coffee consumption, especially since caffeine is an addictive substance. Try cutting out coffee for a week or two, and then see if you need it at all. One of the key concepts of macrobiotics is balance—and addictions are hardly a balanced way of life.

Alcohol

Few nutritionists or health practitioners would advise excessive consumption of alcoholic beverages—or even moderate alcohol consumption on a daily basis. High alcohol consumption has been linked to cirrhosis of the liver, kidney disease, diabetes, fetal alcohol syndrome, mental illness, nervous disorders, and suppression of the immune system. In addition, it's reasonably difficult to maintain overall health—let alone a strong sense of spirituality and more than moderate level of mental acuity—if you're downing highballs after work every day.

But it's possible to drink and still be merry. Even Ohsawa was rumored to take his whiskey neat and on a fairly regular basis—and the macrobiotic diet permits small quantities of sake for drinking and cooking. An occasional—meaning two to four times a week—glass of wine or mug of beer likely won't hurt you unless you're pregnant or have diabetes, kidney problems, liver disorders, or suppression of the immune system, including any viral or bacterial infections. Alcohol should be considered suspect or contraband if you've had previous problems with alcohol or if anyone in your family has a history of alcoholism.

If you choose to drink alcoholic beverages, be aware that not all cocktails are the same. Vodka is a pure distilled grain, with few additives, but other alcoholic beverages, such as whiskey, tequila, gin, and brandy, contain deleterious additives designed to impart flavor. In Germany, where beer purity laws and regulations (which require that beer contain only water, hops, malt, and yeast) are strictly enforced, beer is a simple, natural beverage. In the United States, however, most mass-produced beers contain chemical additives to enhance flavor, color, texture, and foaming. Specialty brews that are virtually unprocessed and approach the levels of purity established in Germany are now available from microbreweries and some larger brewers.

Wine became a much maligned beverage several years ago, as considerable media attention and often unfounded controversy surrounded the issue of sulfites. Sulfites occur naturally in foods and are generally not harmful in small amounts, except to a few people who are sensitive to them. However, additional sulfites are added to wine as a preservative, and commercially produced wines contain high concentrations of herbicide and pesticide residues from the grape-growing process. Organic wines are now available, and while they still contain small amounts of naturally occurring sulfites, they're free of chemical pesticides and additional sulfites used as preservatives. Small amounts of wine and sake can be helpful—and healthful—in cooking, allowing creative chefs to use less oil in everything from braised greens to sautéed shrimp.

One more point to consider: A number of studies suggest that one cocktail a day may actually promote overall health. In 1993 *The Lancet* published a report from the University of California at Davis about the heart-protective effects of phenols from red wines. It appears that red wine offers seven times the antioxidant, heart-protective power of vitamin E. Protective compounds in red wine occur at five times the concentration of those in white wine. A Kaiser Permanente study of 300,000 Californians found that among those who consumed alcohol, wine drinkers (especially red-wine drinkers) had the lowest risk of heart disease. Researchers hypothesized that phenols contained in red wine, especially resveratrol, quercetin, and epicatechin, help to prevent low-density lipoprotein (LDL) cholesterol from becoming oxidized and to reduce the occurrence of arterial plaque.

More research suggests that a drink a day of any kind of alcohol may actually be beneficial to cardiovascular health. A 1994 study at Brigham and Women's Hospital in Boston found that one or two drinks a day may protect against the formation of blood clots that lead to heart attacks. The researchers noted that there is extensive evidence that mortality is reduced in those who consume one or two drinks a day, but that consumption of three or more drinks a day is associated with increased mortality.

Liquids

Ohsawa recommended consuming no more than three or four cups of liquid a day—one of his main principles of the macrobiotic diet was keeping liquids to a minimum. The modern rationale behind this mandate is that a diet high in fresh vegetables, grains, and legumes provides more liquid content than a diet high in processed foods. And while cooking with salt tends to make foods more yang (less yin, or "drier"), the addition of small amounts of fruit and some raw vegetables in the daily diet will provide additional water for the body. Liquids are extremely yin, and it is believed that most health problems and diseases are the result of excessive yin imbalances. Ohsawa believed that a diet that includes relatively small amounts of water and other liquid is more yang and generally more healthful, but traditional macrobiotic practitioners continue to recognize the need for adequate liquids in the diet.

Whether or not you choose to follow the formula for limited amounts of liquid, as mandated by the macrobiotic regimen, there is one macrobiotic rule that should be strictly followed: Meals—macro or otherwise—should be eaten without beverages, since excess liquid intake tends to dilute stomach acids, making digestion more difficult and inhibiting the assimilation of nutrients.

Liquids used in the macrobiotic diet include mineral, spring, and well water; amazake; soy milk; rice milk; bancha tea; green tea; roasted-grain coffee substitutes; Mu tea; and, occasionally, umeboshi plum tea—all served without honey. Fruit juices are generally avoided, since they're highly concentrated forms of fruit (it generally takes three to four oranges to make one cup of juice) and are excessively yin in quality. Coffee, black tea, and carbonated beverages are excluded as well. Japanese customs hold that small amounts of alcoholic beverages before the meal help stimulate the appetite and aid digestion. So have a cup of sake if you are so inclined, but drink it in moderation. (This macrobiotic maxim obviously applies to evening meals—sake is generally ill-advised for breakfast.)

Grain beverages and most macrobiotic teas have a unique woody or nutty taste, and while they admittedly take some getting used to—especially if you have a pampered palate accustomed to coffee with cream and several spoonfuls of sugar—if you start drinking them on a regular basis, you may wonder how you could have imbibed the bitter, black brew we call coffee before breakfast. But be realistic, and don't expect this to happen overnight.

Teas used in the macrobiotic diet come from a variety of sources. Bancha, kukicha, green, and black teas are all harvested from the same plant—the tea bush, which grows in China, Japan, India, and other parts of Asia. However, the teas vary depending on the portions of the plant that are used (buds, leaves, twigs, or stems), the season in which they are harvested, and the processing procedures used. Green tea, a mild stimulant with antibacterial qualities, has long been thought to have health-inducing properties. Studies in Japan have pointed to lower rates of lung cancer, stomach cancer, and skin tumors and lower cholesterol levels among those who drink green tea every day. Research from the National Cancer Institute indicates that green tea may help reduce the incidence of cancer of the esophagus.

Most herbal teas, such as peppermint or chamomile, are avoided in the traditional macrobiotic diet, because these and other herbs, by their nature, have medicinal properties. On the same principle that you wouldn't capriciously consume antibiotics and aspirin, herbal teas shouldn't be consumed on a regular basis, unless you're trying to cure a specific malady. But this

Bancha

Bancha is one of the most popular macrobiotic teas. It's derived from the leaves, stems, or twigs of the tea bush and is harvested in late summer or fall, when the caffeine has receded from the plant. The roasting procedure renders the tea virtually free of caffeine and tannic acid. Bancha tea is sometimes mistakenly called kukicha tea, which is actually made from the twigs of the three-year-old plant and is an entirely different tea. All bancha tea is alkaline in quality, and may be served plain or with a spoonful of brown rice syrup or barley malt syrup.

Green tea

Green tea is harvested in the spring from the young green leaves of the tea bush. It has a slightly bitter taste and is higher in caffeine than bancha. Green tea can be mixed with bancha tea to tone down the bitter flavor.

Black tea

Higher in caffeine and tannic acid, black tea is made from the leaves of the tea bush; the leaves are

rule can, of course, generally be bent without undue detrimental consequences to your health.

You probably don't need to gulp down two quarts of liquid a day if you're consuming mostly whole foods with a relatively high water content. But until your diet is firmly established in the whole-foods arena, decrease liquids gradually. Once you've reached the elusive but obtainable pinnacle of success where most of your diet consists of whole grains, vegetables, and legumes, don't feel compelled to drink like a camel crossing the Sahara. Just listen to your body—it will tell you when it's thirsty. And when it says it's thirsty, drink.

WATER

Water is required for the body's metabolic reactions. When the body becomes dehydrated, metabolism slows down and electrolyte imbalances can occur, leading to nervous disorders and a substantial decrease in energy levels. Water is essential for numerous bodily functions: It's the major component of blood and contains much dissolved oxygen, which is easily assimilated by the body; it helps prevent constipation; it flushes the body of metabolic wastes; and it stimulates liver and kidney function.

In Oriental practices—and in modern orthodox medicine—the kidneys are considered one of the cornerstones of health. Ohsawa believed that when the kidneys malfunction, the body becomes tired and lethargic, and overall health is diminished. Under the macrobiotic philosophy, liquid consumption should be only enough so that urination occurs twice a day for women and three times a day for men. Modern thought holds that water is essential to "flush" toxins from the kidneys. According to Ohsawa, this commonly accepted conclusion is egregiously erroneous in its assumption that the kidneys are "similar in structure and function to a mechanical sewage system. . . . The kidney, however, is not a cast iron pipe. It contains tissue that must be flexible and porous so that the processes of filtration, diffusion and reabsorption can take place."

Most nutritionists and health practitioners today advise drinking one to two quarts of water a day. While this dictum contradicts macrobiotic principles, in practice neither approach is entirely accurate. Differences in climate and environment, living habits, and levels of activity make strict mandates on water consumption ill advised. More liquid intake is advantageous, if not crucial, in dry climates. Water is used for hydrolysis of protein, so if you increase your intake of protein foods, your level of water consumption should increase accordingly. If you smoke cigarettes or drink alcohol, water can help move these extra metabolic wastes through the body and lessen the burden on the kidneys and liver. In addition, high levels of physical and mental activity and excessive stress increase the body's requirement for water.

A Warning About Water

Just because it's clear doesn't mean it's clean. Don't trust your municipal water supply, and forget about turning on the tap, even for cooking. Federal and state standards for drinking water safety are generally grossly inadequate, and known cancer-causing agents exist in almost all municipal water supplies. Most contain chemical additives like chlorine, pesticide residues, nitrates, detergents, and heavy metals. The macrobiotic diet recommends natural spring water or deep-well water for cooking and drinking, but even well waters may be suspect. Hard waters, which have a higher mineral content, are recommended for drinking and cooking.

While tap water is generally free of bacteria and parasites that will make you ill immediately, purification procedures used in municipal water-treatment plants don't remove pollutants that have long-term effects on health. If you think you're safe drinking directly from the kitchen sink just because you don't live near areas with known polluters, think again. Your tap water may contain toxins and pollutants from other nearby areas or from water pipes within and outside your house.

There are five main types of pollutants present in most sources of water.

1. *Microorganisms.* Bacteria, viruses, and parasites may be present in municipal water supplies. Most bacteria and parasites are virtually eliminated by chlorine, but viruses are much more difficult to remove and may be present in varying amounts in tap water.
2. *Toxic minerals.* Aluminum, arsenic, asbestos, barium, chromium, fluoride, nitrate, and toxins such as cadmium, lead, and mercury are found in municipal sources of treated tap water. These inorganic minerals naturally occur in water in small amounts, but pollution from mining and agricultural practices can greatly increase their levels in drinking water.
3. *Organic chemicals.* Animal wastes, fertilizers, pesticides, herbicides, paints, fuels, plastics, and dyes may be present in municipal water supplies. Recent research has detected the presence of harmful chemicals created when chlorine in water treatment procedures combines with organic substances, forming chlorinated carbons (that is, chloroform).
4. *Radioactive substances.* Uranium and radioactive gases such as radon occur naturally in small amounts in many sources of water, but hospitals and many manufacturing operations, including pharmaceutical companies and biomedical research institutes, often dump low-level radioactive wastes into sewers, which find their way into public water supplies.
5. *Additives.* Municipal water-treatment facilities add chemicals, mainly chlorine that is sometimes combined with ammonia, to the water

fermented and highly processed. Dozens of varieties of black tea are available. Oolong tea, for example, is made from a combination of black and green tea leaves and may be flavored with jasmine.

Roasted grain beverages

Roasted barley tea and roasted brown rice tea have mild, nutty flavors and are recommended for daily use. They may be mixed with bancha or green teas and can be served with a small amount of sweetener. You can make them at home or purchase them in natural-products stores and some supermarkets.

Mu tea

Traditionally used for medicinal purposes, Mu tea is prepared from either nine or sixteen herbs, including ginseng, and is a strong, slightly sweet brew. The nine-herb formula contains ginseng, peony root, Japanese parsley root, hoelen, cinnamon, licorice, peach kernels, ginger, and rhemmania. In addition to these nine herbs, the sixteen-herb formula contains seven other herbs: mandarin orange peel, cnicus, atractylis, cypress, cloves, moutan, and coptis. Unless you have access to a natural-products store with a truly exemplary bulk herb section, you won't be able to find most of these herbs. Mu tea is, however, available prepackaged at natural-products stores and Oriental markets.

Coffee substitutes

Most coffee substitutes are prepared from chicory and roasted grains such as barley, brown rice, and wheat. You can make them at home, but a wide variety is available in natural-products stores. If you're trying to kick a coffee habit with grain coffee substitutes, start off by serving them with a little rice or soy milk and a spoonful of barley malt syrup. Supermarket brands of coffee substitutes generally contain high quantities of sweeteners, so check the labels.

Umeboshi tea

Often used for medicinal purposes, umeboshi tea is made from boiling umeboshi plums. It may be served warm or at room temperature and is generally taken without sweeteners.

during the purification process. Fluoride—derived from the toxic gas fluorine—is also added to most municipal water supplies. Flocculents, which make pollutants clump together for more efficient removal in the filtering process, are also added. And even though the Environmental Protection Agency (EPA) classifies some flocculents as probable human carcinogens, it still allows their use in water-treatment facilities.

Bottled waters seem to be the easiest and most convenient alternative to tap water. But not all bottled waters are equal in terms of purity and relative health value. The term *drinking water* may be a meaningless and misleading merchandising term and is not indicative of the quality of the water—so-called "drinking water," in some cases, is nothing more than bottled tap water. For the macrobiotic diet, spring water is generally preferred.

With the number of readily available options for water—ranging from carbon filtration to distillation processes—there's no reason to use drinking and cooking water that isn't perfectly suited to your needs and your level of convenience and commitment. Filtration and purification processes are wildly disparate in terms of their levels of effectiveness and efficiency. During the purification process, some systems remove minerals thought to be beneficial while at the same time removing detrimental microorganisms and toxins. Other systems are ineffective in removing heavy metals. The most common purification methods, some of which can be used at home, are distillation, reverse osmosis, sediment filtration, carbon filtration, and filtration using membrane and ceramic filters..

In the distillation process, water is evaporated by heating; it is then cooled and condensed back into liquid form, leaving behind dissolved matter and heavy metals. The resulting water is extremely pure, but since about 99 percent of all dissolved matter in water is composed of minerals, the resulting liquid is virtually mineral free, rendering it less nutritionally valuable and flat tasting. Distilled water is not recommended in the macrobiotic diet. Since minerals have been almost completely removed from the water, distilled water may leach minerals from the body. And because the distillation procedure uses electricity, it's a costly, energy-intensive, and decidedly cumbersome procedure.

The reverse osmosis procedure relies on extremely high water pressure—generally at a level of forty pounds per square inch—to force water molecules through a fine filter membrane, which removes high concentrations of minerals. While it's far more effective than most filtration and purification methods, especially when combined with carbon filtration, the reverse osmosis system is generally inefficient and expensive. The purification process is extremely slow and energy-intensive, and about eight gallons of untreated water are required to produce one gallon of purified water. Reverse osmosis systems are not as effective in removing contaminants as distillation procedures.

Sediment filtration methods use screens to remove dirt and other particles from the water. Municipal water systems use sediment filters to remove large, coarse particles of contaminants, but this method is ineffective in removing chemicals, heavy metals, bacteria, parasites, and harmful microorganisms.

The use of carbon is one of the most popular home filtration methods and is reasonably effective in removing organic chemicals, chlorine, chloroform, and radon, eliminating an estimated 80–99 percent of these toxins. But carbon cannot remove microorganisms or toxic minerals and can actually be a breeding ground for bacteria if filters are changed infrequently. Two types of carbon filters are used: block and granulated. Block carbon is more effective, but it also requires a sediment filter. If you choose to use carbon filters for home water purification systems, the two primary considerations are the length of time the filter is in contact with the water (obviously, the longer the better) and the need to change the filter often, which requires a certain level of attention and commitment.

Membrane and ceramic filters are designed to specifically remove bacteria and parasites. Ceramic filters are longer lasting and sturdier than membrane filters.

Tropical Fruits

Excessive fruit consumption, especially of fruits from tropical climates, is generally discouraged in the traditional macrobiotic program because it's extremely yin, and most disease is thought to be of yin origin. But there are exceptions to every rule. Temperate fruits are permitted in moderate quantities, and if you live in a warm climate, bananas and mangos are more than acceptable. Even in colder climates, most fruits are included in small quantities on a daily or semiweekly basis, depending on the season.

So, dare you eat a peach? The answer is, of course, yes—but go a little lighter on the mangos. The complete exclusion of all fruit is neither necessary nor advisable. Fruit contains simple carbohydrates and easily assimilated nutrients and enzymes, and it is healthful on a number of fronts. Apples in particular contain high concentrations of pectin and other fibers, which have been shown to lower rates of colon cancer. If you include fruit in your daily diet, it should be raw, fresh, and whole in order to provide the highest degree of nutritional value and fiber. Generally, dried fruits are used more freely than fresh fruits in the macrobiotic diet, since the drying process is thought to diminish excess water, or yin energy.

Some schools of thought maintain that fruit is the ideal food for breakfast, when you probably haven't eaten for eight to ten hours, since it's easily assimilated and provides a ready source of energy. Fruit should be eaten at least three to four hours after or thirty minutes before meals, and it should never be consumed with protein sources because the combination of protein and fruit sugars slows the digestive process and can cause food to be detained in the stomach for up to eight hours. Some believe this dictum is especially true for tropical fruits.

RAW VERSUS COOKED FOODS

The idea behind eating raw foods is to maintain a balance between cooked and uncooked foods and to take the climate, the season, and your individual body makeup into account. Raw foods are generally consumed in somewhat limited quantities in the traditional macrobiotic diet. Cooking is one of the first steps in the digestion and assimilation of foods. It helps break down tough cellulose walls and makes nutrients more bioavailable to the body. Other macrobiotic foods served without heating are still, in the strictest sense of the word, "cooked"—pickling, for example, breaks down cellulose walls and begins the process of metabolizing proteins.

Proponents of the raw-food diet maintain that enzymes are the crucial contributors to overall health. Enzymes are naturally occurring substances that are catalysts for metabolic activities and that aid biochemical processes in the body. Three types of enzymes are necessary for metabolism: proteolytic enzymes or proteases to break down protein, lipolytic enzymes or lipases to break down fat, and amylolytic enzymes or amylases to break down carbohydrates. It is believed that a lack of these enzymes in the digestive system inhibits proper absorption of food and allows toxins to accumulate in the colon. Foods are the primary sources of enzymes, and raw-food-diet proponents hold that cooking destroys enzymes, denaturing the structure of protein molecules, destroying related enzymes necessary for uptake and absorption, and rendering food effectively "dead." An interesting concept, to be sure, but not one that is necessarily nutritionally or scientifically valid.

The raw-foods dictums are by no means in direct contradiction to macrobiotic principles. There is very little scientific proof that enzymes are absorbed intact from raw food. Many vitamins and phytochemical compounds are heat-stable. Cooking may, indeed, free up some compounds, thus making them more bioavailable. In addition, cooking is not the only way to kill an enzyme. Excess acidity in the stomach also destroys the effectiveness of enzymes—a concept closely aligned with the macrobiotic maxim that most illness results from excess yin, or acid, conditions. The macrobiotic diet advocates carefully cooked foods, as well as methods, such as light steaming and quick sautéing, that preserve the maximum amount of enzymes and other nutrients. Cooking food doesn't mean boiling vegetables to within an inch of their enzymatic lives. You'll never find flaccid broccoli or limp, gray asparagus spears in a properly prepared macrobiotic meal.

Sprouts are used in the macrobiotic diet—and rather extensively in the meal plans in this book—as an easily digested form of raw food with a high enzyme content (sprouting techniques are reviewed on page 88). Fermented foods such as miso and tempeh contain a relatively high level of enzymes yielded by the activity of beneficial bacteria in the fermenting process.

7

GETTING REAL

NOW THAT YOU KNOW WHAT YOU'RE SUPPOSED TO DO according to the principles of a macrobiotic diet, here's the big question: Who's going to provide you with an extra seven hours a day to make soup stocks and sprout alfalfa seeds? Not to worry. A plethora of painless methods exists to make planning and preparation easier.

It's an immutable fact that most people simply don't have the time, energy, or inclination to devote three or four hours a day to food planning and preparation. Although fresh fruits and vegetables purchased the day you plan to use them are the ideal, there will be more than a few occasions when frequent forays to the grocery store are beyond your capabilities. The short cuts that follow can help you become realistic about unavoidable limitations.

A variety of canned and frozen foods are available in natural-products stores—they're fine for occasional use and infinitely preferable to a stop at the fast-food drive-through. Even though freshly prepared foods are unarguably superior, making large quantities of your own dishes at home and then refrigerating or freezing them to use later in the week is more than acceptable. So unless you're trying to cure a particular disease, bending the rules and still adhering to a generally healthy diet is far more beneficial to your mental and physical health than tossing up your hands in despair and calling out for MSG-laden Chinese delivery because you don't have three hours to boil barley just before serving.

Breakfast and Lunch on the Go

The traditional American breakfast repast generally consists of food that's high in fat and sugar—consider the ubiquitous Danish—and that jolts the body into a hyperalert but artificial state of awareness, shocking sleepy nerves, sending the adrenals into overdrive, and asking far too much from a lethargic digestive system that's been in repose for eight hours or more. In traditional macrobiotic diets, miso soup or suimono, a thin, clear broth, was the first meal of the day. It efficiently increased the body's depleted glucose levels and gently roused the stomach into action.

If you've already decided that soup isn't the solution to breaking your fast, an abundance of options nonetheless exists. Obviously, bacon and cheese omelets aren't up for consideration—at least not on a daily basis—and the Danish or doughnut equivalents are less-than-viable alternatives, macrobiotic or not. Since yeast-containing foods are generally avoided on the macro regimen, bagels and other breads aren't recommended for everyday use.

If the thought of soup scattered with bits of floating seaweed doesn't strike you as the ideal meal before noon, you can still partake of and not forsake the traditional macrobiotic ideals. Brown rice is commonly served in the traditional macrobiotic diet as a breakfast food, and countless variations on this theme are possible. Grain-based dishes are ideal breakfast foods. They provide complex carbohydrates for energy that will last for hours, they're easily digested, and they're fast and convenient—especially with the creative and resourceful use of leftovers. A grain-based breakfast doesn't have to consist of a bowl of dry brown rice and a pair of chopsticks.

In warm-weather months leftover brown rice (or millet, barley, or bulghur) makes a tasty morning meal served cold with rice or soy milk and sliced fresh fruits. When the weather is cooler, a variety of grains left over from the night before can be heated with soy milk; sprinkled with dried fruits, nuts, and seeds; and sweetened with brown rice syrup for a hearty meal. Toss in a handful of oats, processed briefly in a food mill, to thicken the mixture and give it a creamy texture, and try adding a little vanilla or cinnamon for flavor (see the recipes for these and other breakfast quickies in chapter 16).

Leftover grains can also be mixed with whole-grain flour, soy milk, and a handful of nuts or seeds to make pancakes—called *okonomi* in Japanese cookery—with terrific textures. Serve them with maple syrup or barley malt syrup in cold weather or with sliced fruit and soy yogurt in the summer. Try cooking them extra thin; spread with tahini or sunflower butter and brown rice syrup, and roll them up for breakfast to go. Unleavened breads spread with nut butters and berry preserves are a fast and simple morning meal as well.

If you live in a warm climate, or if the weather is truly tropical, you may choose to start your day with fruit. While it's not recommended on a daily basis in most macrobiotic practices, fruit is a fast and easy source of energy for a sleepy body. In spring and fall, modest portions of apples, peaches, pears, and grapes may be consumed. Melons make an exemplary morning meal on occasion, but eat them alone, not mixed with other fruits or protein foods.

In the hottest months of summer, a smoothie made with rice or soy milk, berries, and a small amount of banana (skip the ice—it's too harsh on your digestive system first thing in the morning) and sweetened with brown rice syrup is a gentle, easy way to wake up a sluggish metabolism. Or serve a mixture of sliced fruit drizzled with dairy-free yogurt and sprinkled with sesame seeds. Even in the coldest months, temperate climate fruits may be consumed every other day or so, but they are best served warm. Try applesauce, baked apples, pear and berry compotes, or apricot or peach crunches.

Vegetables can also be incorporated into breakfast—winter squash left over from the night before can be mashed and stirred into millet for a porridge or blended with a little tahini or sunflower butter for a spread on unleavened bread. Baked root vegetables rewarmed in a small pan with a little barley malt syrup and sunflower seeds make an unusual but tasty breakfast—the barley malt syrup brings out the natural sweetness of the roots. Don't use root vegetables that have been prepared with garlic, black pepper, and roasted sesame oil—they obviously don't mix well with grain sweeteners.

PLANNING AHEAD: DECREASING PREPARATION TIME

Almost everything you'll prepare from the recipe section in this book takes about twenty minutes. But some recipes require a little advance preparation, especially those that use sprouted ingredients, stocks, beans, and some types of grains, and there will be times when you won't feel like opening a cookbook to make a simple meal. There are some basic ways to decrease preparation time for the recipes in this book, with ideas designed to spark your creativity for making the most of cooked leftovers and more.

Take Two: Creative Leftovers

One of the best time-savers is the ubiquitous leftover meal. Leftovers are a fact of life, and while the macrobiotic maxim holds that foods should ideally be prepared fresh before each meal, this is a rigorous sentiment not practical in busy lives. Even the Japanese make frequent use of *ojiya,* a traditional dish concocted from leftover rice and soup cooked into a porridge. The judicious and creative use of certain leftovers can be an invaluable time-saver, and it doesn't mean you have to serve the same meal six days running. Some of the following suggestions may sound a little bizarre at first, but have faith and try them out—you'll be more than pleasantly surprised at the results.

Try pureeing leftover soups and stews for sauces, adding fresh herbs for seasoning, and serve the sauce hot over quick-cooking noodles or tossed with leftover grains for cold salads. Thicken pureed stews with a little arrowroot, add pepitas or pine nuts for texture, and fashion them into hearty pancakes as a side dish or snack. Mix pureed stews with whole-grain flour, oats, and sunflower or sesame seeds and fry them up as grain burgers. Leftover vegetables and some cold vegetable salads, like cauliflower or squash salads, can be blended into a smooth texture, thinned with soy milk or stock, and cooked as soups—just be aware of the kinds of ingredients and seasonings used in the original salad (those made with delicate leafy greens or prepared with vinegar-based dressings obviously won't work). Leftover vegetables, pureed until very smooth then thinned with soy milk and flavored with a little tahini, make unusual, flavorful sauces for leafy green vegetables or most noodles.

Noodles and Soups on the Run

You can maintain grains as the center of your meal by using noodles, which cook in a fraction of the time it takes to prepare other grains. Even the pickiest palates will be hard pressed to find fault with properly prepared noodle dishes. An enormous variety of whole-grain, dried noodles, made from various grains and fashioned into countless shapes, are available—everything from the traditional macrobiotic soba and udon noodles, ramen, saifun, somen, and maifun noodles to corn, sesame, wheat, quinoa, artichoke, beet, and spinach noodles, which can be rendered into elbows, spaghetti, spirals, shells, twists, and all manner of other shapes and configurations.

In general, when cooking noodles, bring the water to a full boil. For a consummately convenient noodle dish, however, don't even bother boiling water first—place the whole-grain noodles in cold water and then bring them to a boil to allow the noodles to release their starches and yield a soft, creamy texture. Add sea salt, root or aboveground vegetables, tofu or tempeh, gomashio, and dried herbs as the noodles are cooking, and stir in leafy greens, fresh herbs, and wakame or crumbled nori toward the end of cooking. Add a little tahini, miso, tamari, and ginger for an instant sauce and serve in bowls as a simple, one-dish meal. From beginning to end, this style of preparing noodles takes about ten or fifteen minutes.

Don't toss out vegetables languishing in the bottom of the refrigerator at the end of the week. Instead, try preparing your own version of what I call Refrigerator Reincarnations, as long as the ingredients are still fresh and unspoiled. Use everything in the kitchen to make a Sunday dinner meal before you go shopping to restock for the week. In the winter months, concoct a big pot of soup or stew using a variety of vegetables and any leftover cooked beans and grains. For cooling summer salads, stir-fry the last of your vegetables and toss them with rice or noodles, brown rice vinegar, a small amount of barley malt syrup, nuts or seeds, and a little tofu or tempeh.

Sprouts

You can buy sprouts at natural-products stores, but the selection is somewhat limited and they're usually grossly overpriced. Fresh sprouts are vastly superior in taste and nutritional value to the slightly shriveled and often dried-out retail variety. Since they're so simple to make, few compelling reasons exist for buying the overpriced offerings at natural-products stores.

Sprouting is an ongoing endeavor that requires some attention but little effort—it's like watering houseplants but it's easier, especially if you keep your sprouting containers right by the sink where they're staring you in the face every morning. Wash and soak seeds or beans according to the directions in Table 9. Use a one-quart jar with a screen top (you can buy sprouting jars at most natural-products stores, or make your own using a layer of cheesecloth secured around the top of the jar with a rubber band). After the initial soaking period, pour off the soaking water, rinse the seeds or beans, and drain thoroughly. Let the jar rest on its side away from direct sunlight. Rinse and drain them once a day, while you're standing in the kitchen in the morning, waiting for your tea to boil or bread to toast. When they're ready, sprouts provide a fast snack and can be combined with a little dressing and served as an easy salad or side dish. Stirred into soups and grain dishes just before serving, sprouts add crunchy texture and a fresh, green taste.

Stocks

Some of the recipes in this book require homemade stocks—a proposition that may make you wary with visions of fish bones bubbling away while you, chained to the stove, check your wristwatch every thirty minutes. It's true that making stocks takes time, but there are shortcuts that can make preparation nearly painless. The following stocks don't use chicken necks or trout heads, and they are much easier to prepare than your mother may have told you.

Whenever you steam or boil vegetables, save the cooking water and strain it into a large glass jar. Keep the uncooked tops from turnips, carrots, celery, and other vegetables, as well as onion skins and the ends from root vegetables. Start your own culinary compost heap in the refrigerator, storing uncooked vegetable pieces in a tightly covered glass container (don't store leafy green vegetables in the container—they decompose too quickly). Even apples, cucumbers, and mushrooms can be used in a basic stock.

Table 9
SPROUTING TECHNIQUES

SEED/BEAN	AMOUNT	SOAKING TIME	SPROUTING TIME
Alfalfa	1 tablespoon per quart of water	4–6 hours	5–7 days
Fenugreek	2 tablespoons per quart of water	4–6 hours	5–7 days
Radish	1 tablespoon per quart of water	4–6 hours	3–4 days
Lentil	Fill quart jar ¼ full with beans; cover with water	8 hours	2–3 days
Sunflower	Fill quart jar ¼ full with seeds; cover with water	8 hours	2 days
Mung	Fill quart jar ¼ full with beans; cover with water	Overnight	3–4 days

Once a week, use the leftover cooking water and vegetable parts to make a basic light vegetable stock. Use smaller amounts of cruciferous vegetables (cabbage, cauliflower and broccoli) since they impart an overly strong flavor to the stock. Using a small amount of corn oil, sauté the vegetables until soft and add water to cover. Cover with a tight-fitting lid and bring to a boil, then let it simmer for about two hours, while you read the Sunday paper or run out for brunch. Strain and add seasonings if desired. Store half the stock in a large container in the refrigerator, and freeze the rest in small containers, letting them thaw in the refrigerator the night before you plan to use them.

In addition to the light vegetable stock used in many of the recipes in this book, Kombu Dashi—a traditional Japanese stock—is wonderful as a base for most soups or eaten alone as a clear broth. It is often used as the base for simple miso soups, with a few scallions floated on top for garnish (see page 139). While fresh stocks are superior, don't be afraid to use high-quality canned or powdered vegetable stocks if you're facing a culinary crisis.

Beans and Legumes

Beans and legumes can present logistical problems for busy people because of the cooking time involved, but there are a few shortcuts. When cooking beans, make at least twice as much as you need—the extras can be refrigerated or frozen for later use. Also incorporate softer, faster cooking beans like lentils and mung beans into your meal plans, and prepare them first so they can boil away while you prepare the rest of your meal.

The amount of time required for cooking beans varies. Lentils take about half an hour, while garbanzos can take as long as four hours to fully cook (see Table 7, page 66). With the exception of black-eyed peas, lentils, mung beans, and split peas, most beans must be soaked before cooking to shorten their cooking time and increase their digestibility. Place a few strips of kombu in the bottom of the cooking pot to reduce cooking time and make the beans more digestible.

While boiling is the method most Americans use for preparing beans, the shocking method (pages 65–66) shortens the cooking time and greatly increases flavor. Pressure-cooking also considerably reduces cooking time.

Grains

Grains are also somewhat time consuming to prepare, but with a little forethought and advance preparation, you can shorten cooking times and have a ready supply of grains on hand at all times. Most grains can be soaked overnight to shorten cooking times. A strip of kombu added to the cooking water can greatly lessen cooking times, and pressure-cooking is still the fastest route, reducing the cooking time of rice and other grains and yielding a tastier product. It may be tempting to use processed rice and other fast-cooking grains, but they're so nutritionally inferior that it doesn't make sense to sacrifice.

When you cook rice and other grains, always make more than you need—enough for a day or two—to reheat as main or side dishes, serve as breakfast, or use in recipes. Try using more fast-cooking grains, like couscous, millet, corn grits, and bulghur. And rather than buying processed "quick" oats, run regular whole oats or steel-cut oats (also called Scotch oats) through a food mill for a couple of seconds before cooking to shorten their cooking time. For quickie grains, combine one cup bulghur wheat with three cups warm water, stir, and let sit until the water is absorbed and the wheat is moist and fluffy; then refrigerate.

Keep a steady supply of soaked bulghur wheat on hand. It can be made into a simple tabouli, eaten cold with rice milk and raisins for breakfast, mixed with oats and served as a hot cereal, combined with leftover vegetables and a miso-tahini sauce for lunch, tossed in soups, used with leftover vegetables and sunflower seeds as a base for grain burgers, mixed with a handful of nuts and served either warm or cold as a side dish, or added to vegetable and tempeh stir-fries. The possibilities are nearly limitless.

Vegetables

A word of advice here on advance preparation of vegetables: Don't do it. Chopping up large quantities of vegetables before they're to be used tragically compromises their nutritional value and aesthetic appeal. They will turn brown, wilt faster, and lose many essential vitamins and enzymes. Some vegetables, especially root and hardier above-ground vegetables, can be cut an hour or so before using, but don't chop up mounds of carrots the night before you make carrot and corn bisque for a dinner party. And unless you're preparing meals for twenty or more people, the macrobiotic approach to cooking discourages using food processors. The best advice for fast preparation of vegetables is to practice cutting with your knives.

8

EATING OUT AND
ENTERTAINING

ALL THE PRACTICES AND PHILOSOPHIES DISCUSSED SO FAR, as well as the recipes to come, do not by any means exclude the possibility of pleasure in food. At its highest level, food should border on the intoxicating and should gratify appetites on every level, from the physical and mental to the spiritual. This principle, however, does not prescribe a diet based on pure sensory indulgences without thought to how food intake relates to health on all levels, nor does it advocate a regimen based on bland and uninspiring food. The key is balance. There are numerous healthy, guilt-free recipes, designed to accommodate busy lifestyles and discerning palates, that you can serve without disclaimers at dinner parties or proudly tote to potluck barbecues. You can adhere to the general framework of macrobiotic principles while allowing for various lifestyle factors—like eating out and entertaining.

EATING OUT

If you live in a fairly cosmopolitan area and have a variety of restaurants from which to choose, following a tolerably strict macrobiotic diet poses few problems. Japanese and Chinese restaurants are often the best choices, but, unfortunately, both types of fare vary in quality. Many Chinese restaurants use monosodium glutamate (MSG), canned vegetables (especially bamboo shoots and water chestnuts), and commercial sauces manufactured with high quantities of refined salt, sugar, and preservatives. Even if you request an MSG-free meal, the sauces and condiments used in many dishes contain MSG in one form or another, and if you tell your waiter to hold the MSG, it may simply mean that the cook won't sprinkle the offending substance on your food while it's being heated. Soups are especially suspect, since they're prepared in large quantities ahead of time and usually use commercial seasonings and sauces with chemicals and preservatives. Most high-quality Chinese restaurants recognize the American aversion to MSG, however, and provide alternatives on the menu for special diets. Japanese restaurants offer the widest variety of foods recommended on the macrobiotic diet, but you may still have a hard time finding brown rice, since most use sticky, gelatinous white rice as a staple.

You can construct a mostly macro meal in other restaurants, especially if you stick to ethnic cuisine where dairy is generally not used. American restaurants are increasingly following the California lean-cuisine approach to eating, and you'll generally have little trouble finding foods that are compatible with the macrobiotic maxims. High-quality Mexican restaurants now prepare beans without the use of lard, and if you can find one with whole-wheat tortillas and brown rice—an ever-increasing trend—you can concoct a fairly decent meal. Some even offer soy cheese and sour cream alternatives (permissible in small amounts), and most have some sort of seafood meal on the menu. Stick to the simplest dishes—bean burritos or corn tostadas, without sour cream and cheese and with brown rice (if it's available), or grilled white fish and vegetable side dishes. Ask for larger portions of vegetables and brown rice if possible, and avoid the tortilla chips and hot sauce. Indian and Thai restaurants are heavy on the vegetarian end, but many or most of the dishes are high in fat and heavy, hot seasonings. Focus on the rice dishes, vegetables, dosas, chutneys, and dals, and ask if curry, ghee, and hot pepper sauces can be omitted from your food. Ask for breads listed on the menu with the words "roti" or "nan"— they're usually roasted or baked rather than fried.

Some restaurants—Italian, for example—present true challenges in constructing a macro meal, since most of the dishes are swimming in cream or tomato sauces and cheese—but it can be done. Order appetizer-size portions of fish, side dishes of pasta, and extra servings of vegetables. Some sympathetic chefs will even prepare a platter of fresh vegetables. If nothing else is available, stick to a simple salad and pasta tossed with olive oil and herbs. Creole cuisine and Greek, German, and Russian fare are reasonably challenging in terms of constructing a mostly macro meal, and steak houses are generally not feasible for macro fare unless they offer fish dishes as well.

ENTERTAINING

Entertaining on a macro regimen isn't nearly as challenging as it may seem. The recipes in this book are designed to appeal to all palates. For potlucks, choose dishes that go light on the traditional macrobiotic ingredients. You don't want to freak out your friends with inordinate amounts of seaweed and umeboshi plum, but if you choose tempura dishes and tempeh stir-fries, they'll be pleasantly surprised by how tasty macro meals can be. Choose simple, easy-to-prepare dishes and those that can be made ahead of time, so you don't find yourself chained to a pressure cooker during most of the festivities. Pay particular attention to aesthetic details: Present food with creative garnishes, including edible flowers and greens, and incorporate dishes of various textures, colors, and flavors.

Dinner parties are hardly an arduous endeavor, even in the macro realm. A plethora of palatable dishes can be found in the recipe section. These range from the modestly macro to those with a more decidedly ethnic flavor and flair. For a lighter summer meal, try starting with Bitter Greens with Raspberry Poppyseed Vinaigrette and chilled Summer Squash Soup with Pepitas; then serve Shrimp with Cilantro Walnut Pesto as the main course. For a warming winter meal, start with Garbanzo Beet Chapati served with Sprouted Hummus as an appetizer, Green Beans with Burdock and Mirin or Appled Beets as side dishes, and a hearty main course like Wild Mushroom and Barley Stew or Mixed-Bean Polenta.

If you want to go all out and are intent on impressing friends with real, live macro fare—or if you want to try it yourself—throw a traditional macrobiotic dinner party complete with ceremonial dishes such as *Omedeto* (roughly translated to mean "congratulations rice"), *Aemono-aisho-ae* (meaning "harmonious combination"), and *Kinton*, a traditional dessert made by blending equal parts cooked chestnuts and steamed or baked sweet potatoes. Other traditional ceremonial dishes served on holidays and for special occasions include deep-fried lotus root, strips of boiled kombu tied in knots and served with dipping sauces, and mochi with azuki beans, apple, raisins, almonds, and tamari.

While desserts aren't a standard part of the macrobiotic diet, they can be used on occasion and don't need to be decadent to be delicious. Pies and tarts prepared with whole-wheat crust and fresh, temperate climate fruits make marvelous summer desserts, served warm with rice or soy ice-cream alternatives. Stewed fruit topped with a mixture of pureed tofu, almond butter, and rice syrup is a warming and flavorful finish to a winter meal. Millet porridges with nuts or seeds and winter squashes pureed into puddings with silken tofu and grain sweeteners are perfect desserts. *Shiruko*, a traditional dessert made of azuki beans that are cooked until very soft and served with baked mochi, is a wonderfully healthy end to any meal.

A variety of cookies and cakes can be prepared without yeast using whole-grain flours, barley malt syrup or brown rice syrup, dried fruits and nuts, and soy milk. You don't even have to tell your guests they're eating macrobiotic food. They may never figure it out.

ON THE ROAD

If you've chosen to follow a fairly strict macrobiotic diet, eating while traveling can be a Herculean task at best. Flying generally presents fewer dietary dilemmas, since travel time is short and special meals are available. The sanest advice, unless you're flying first class, is to avoid airline food altogether, but if this is out of the question, order special meals. The vegetarian varieties are execrable and generally contain refined white flour and dairy. The vegan and macrobiotic meals offered by some airlines aren't even worth describing. Order seafood meals instead, which generally consist of three or four boiled shrimp, about a tablespoon of salmon, sometimes a small portion of pasta or even soba noodles, green salad, and whole-grain bread—about as close to macrobiotic as you'll get at 35,000 feet.

Those who have attempted to take road trips while eschewing meat, dairy, refined grains, and canned vegetables know the rigors and risks involved. Having consumed thousands of bowls of oatmeal and over-cooked green beans in roadside cafés during cross-country jaunts, I have found ways to travel and still generally stick to the principles of the macrobiotic diet. Even the most appalling truck stops and neon-lit diners with linoleum decor generally offer oatmeal for breakfast. The on-the-road version of macrobiotic lunches and dinners will generally consist of vegetables and rice—whole grain, if providence prevails—and fish, which is recommended only if you're within walking distance of open waters. If you are blessed with a kind and patient waitress, explain your dilemma and ask for a steamed vegetable plate—hopefully, they'll have something relatively green that hasn't been boiled with ham hocks.

As far as fast-food restaurants go, don't expect to find anything that adheres to macrobiotic mandates. You'll be able to find meat-free dishes, a modicum of dairy-free offerings, and a few so-called salads (generally consisting of a pile of watery iceberg lettuce and pale pink tomatoes) but little else. Even this vegetarian fare is prepared and served with low-grade fats and lots of sodium. Find a supermarket instead, or look for a convenience store, where you'll at least be able to find sunflower seeds, raisins, apples, and, if you're truly blessed, whole-grain crackers and air-popped popcorn.

Your best bet is to be a good cub scout and travel prepared. Leave room in the back seat of your car for a large cooler and stock up at the store before you leave home. Buy temperate-climate fruits (apples, pears, and peaches), dried fruits, nuts and seeds, individual servings of soy or rice milk, small bags of unsweetened granola, rice cakes, tahini, barley malt syrup or brown rice syrup, and packaged baked tofu. Prepare grains and beans ahead of time and pack them in well-sealed containers, either plain or seasoned and mixed with vegetables. Take along some miso and gomashio as well as a little wakame or hijiki. I have often traveled with tiny Tupperware containers of miso and plastic bags of seaweed in my purse, asked at the greasiest-spoon restaurants for a small pot of hot water and an empty bowl, and concocted miso soup with wakame right in my linoleum booth, much to the horror and perverse delight of my fellow diners. Of course, I always leave a tip.

9

A MONTH OF MACRO
Daily Meal Plans

THE FOLLOWING MEAL PLANS were devised to incorporate mostly macrobiotic principles, with the inclusion of miso on a daily basis and small amounts of seaweed and sprouts several times a week. These meals are suitable for temperate climates and seasons—adjustments should be made for hotter and colder times of the year. For example, miso soup can be eaten cool or at room temperature during the summer, and cold grain salads may be heated in the winter months.

Dishes that begin with capital letters are included in the recipe section of this book; the others are self-explanatory. Asterisks are included when extra portions of the listed food or dish should be prepared for use in a dish the following day. (This doesn't mean you should shy away from one-day-old leftovers—if dinner the night before was spectacular, by all means enjoy it for lunch the next day. Just don't let leftovers go for more than a day or so.) Beverages should not be consumed with meals, with the exception of small quantities of kukicha or bancha tea at breakfast.

WEEK ONE
Monday
Breakfast: rice cream with almonds, raisins, and soy milk
Lunch: Fried Soba Noodles; miso soup with shiitake and arame

Dinner: Tempeh and Burdock with Red Pepper Puree; steamed kale* with sesame seeds and brown rice vinegar; brown rice*

Tuesday

Breakfast: whole-grain cereal, almond or soy milk; baked apple with brown rice syrup

Lunch: Brown Rice Salad with Sesame Ginger Sauce; mellow white miso soup with scallions and kale

Dinner: Broccoli and Wild Rice* Pancakes; steamed or fried tofu* with Mushroom Gravy; Watercress Beets with Walnuts

Wednesday

Breakfast: oatmeal with almonds, raisins, and rice milk; mochi with tahini and honey

Lunch: Sunny Tofu Salad on pita; miso soup with broccoli and wild rice

Dinner: Rosemary Winter Squash Stew; Bitter Greens with Raspberry Poppyseed Vinaigrette; buckwheat* with corn and pine nuts

Thursday

Breakfast: buckwheat (hot or cold) with rice milk and blueberries; mochi with tahini and honey

Lunch: seitan and mixed-vegetable stir-fry; miso kombu broth; flat bread

Dinner: udon noodles* with leeks and peas; Honey Carrots* with Caraway Seeds; boiled lentils* with arame

Friday

Breakfast: millet porridge with apricots, almonds, and rice milk

Lunch: udon noodle sushi rolls and slivered Honey Carrots with Caraway Seeds; miso soup with wakame and lentils

Dinner: tempeh stir-fried with shiitakes and snow peas; barley;* steamed watercress* and beets*

Saturday

Breakfast: stewed fruit compote with Almond Cream; mochi

Lunch: barley salad with carrots, beets, and sprouted azuki beans; Creamy Watercress Soup (hot or cold)

---

* Starred reference indicates that you should make extra for meals the next day.

Dinner: Ginger Plum Scallops; short-grain brown rice* with sesame seeds; Braised Radicchio and Currants

Sunday

Breakfast: brown rice pancakes with Apple Raisin Syrup; blueberries and rice milk

Lunch: Hearty Corn and Asparagus Stir-Fry; endive and chicory salad* with sprouted azuki beans; miso soup with ginger and mushrooms

Dinner: Refrigerator Reincarnations (see page 87 for instructions)

WEEK TWO

Monday

Breakfast: sweet potatoes with Apple Raisin Syrup; rice milk; flat bread

Lunch: Egg-Less Salad pita sandwich with alfalfa sprouts; braised endive and chicory salad; miso soup with scallions and burdock

Dinner: corn* and mushrooms stir-fried with tempeh; buckwheat;* steamed collard greens* with sesame seeds

Tuesday

Breakfast: bulghur wheat (hot or cold) with rice milk, dried apricots, and raisins

Lunch: Corn and Buckwheat Crunch; cold braised greens with brown rice vinegar; miso soup with carrots, mushrooms, and daikon

Dinner: seitan stir-fried with leeks and red peppers; Brussels sprouts;* whole-wheat couscous

Wednesday

Breakfast: couscous with rice milk; stewed fruit compote

Lunch: Brussels sprouts salad with grated carrots, arame, and Peanut Ginger Dressing; miso kombu broth; flat bread

Dinner: tempeh stir-fried with mustard greens and summer squash; quinoa* with pepitas; pinto beans*

Thursday

Breakfast: corn flakes with raisins and rice milk; mochi

---

* Starred reference indicates that you should make extra for meals the next day.

Lunch: Crunchy Quinoa Salad with pinto beans; miso soup with scallions and ginger

Dinner: Baked Tofu, Shallots, and Wild Mushrooms; black beans with cilantro;* steamed asparagus;* soba noodles

Friday

Breakfast: millet porridge with rice milk and pecans

Lunch: Asparagus and Yellow Pepper Toss with soba noodles; miso soup with black beans and shiitake mushrooms

Dinner: seitan stir-fried with tamari and Swiss chard;* Parsnip Puree; steamed brown rice*

Saturday

Breakfast: baked apples with raisins and rice syrup

Lunch: nori seitan rolls with rice and Swiss chard; miso soup with scallions and ginger

Dinner: Tempeh* and Celery Hearts with Mustard Tahini Sauce; corn noodles;* steamed mixed vegetables*

Sunday

Breakfast: oatmeal with raisins and rice milk; apple (raw or baked)

Lunch: corn noodles (hot or cold) with chopped mixed vegetables and tempeh; miso kombu broth with arame

Dinner: Refrigerator Reincarnations (see page 87 for instructions)

WEEK THREE

Monday

Breakfast: flat bread with Tahini Apple Butter; stewed fruit with dried apricots

Lunch: Sprouted Hummus with alfalfa sprouts and pita bread; miso and kombu broth

Dinner: Summer Squash Soup with Pepitas (hot or cold—winter squash may be substituted); fried tempeh* with onions and collard greens;* boiled udon noodles* with tamari

---

* Starred reference indicates that you should make extra for meals the next day.

Tuesday

Breakfast: fruit compote; rice milk and corn flakes

Lunch: tempeh sandwich with sprouts; miso soup with udon noodles and collard greens

Dinner: Roots* and Greens Casserole; Belgian endive salad and pine nuts with Creamy Ginger Dressing; brown and wild rice*

Wednesday

Breakfast: baked root vegetables with brown rice syrup, raisins, and cinnamon; mochi

Lunch: Wild Side Salad; miso soup with burdock and dulse

Dinner: tofu, carrots, and spinach stir-fry; barley* with almonds; black beans;* Garbanzo Beet Chapati*

Thursday

Breakfast: barley (hot or cold) with Blueberry Sauce

Lunch: Black Bean Soup with Roasted Red Peppers; green salad with sprouts; Poppyseed Onion Chapati

Dinner: seitan stir-fried with daikon and collard greens;* whole-wheat couscous;* baked squash (summer or winter);* miso kombu broth

Friday

Breakfast: baked squash (hot or cold) with barley malt syrup; oats with rice milk

Lunch: couscous salad with sprouted beans, seitan, daikon, and collard greens; miso soup with mushrooms and scallions

Dinner: Roasted Pepper Casserole with Cilantro Millet* Custard (make extra millet separately); chicory, arugula, and radicchio salad;* sesame noodles* tossed with cumin and olive oil

Saturday

Breakfast: cold millet with raspberries and rice milk; mochi with tahini and honey

Lunch: sesame noodles with sprouted beans, chicory, arugula, radicchio, and Creamy Ginger Dressing (hot or cold); miso soup with scallions

Dinner: Cinnamon Sole;* Red Peppers in Mirin;* Wild Rice* Pesto

---

* Starred reference indicates that you should make extra for meals the next day.

Sunday

Breakfast: pancakes with wild rice and Blueberry Sauce

Lunch: Belgian Endive and Burdock; sushi rolls with sole and sprouts; miso kombu broth

Dinner: Refrigerator Reincarnations (see page 87 for instructions)

WEEK FOUR

Monday

Breakfast: oatmeal with dried apricots, rice milk, and brown rice syrup; apple (baked or raw)

Lunch: steamed collard greens and tofu; miso soup with vegetable noodles

Dinner: tempeh stir-fried with bok choy and shiitakes; mixed boiled beans (azukis, black beans, mung beans, lentils, navy beans, pinto beans, peas); short-grain brown rice*

Tuesday

Breakfast: brown rice (hot or cold) with raisins and rice milk

Lunch: Seven-Bean Salad with Creamy Ginger Dressing; miso kombu broth

Dinner: Wild Mushroom and Barley Stew; Cauliflower Millet* Mash (prepare extra millet separately); steamed spinach*

Wednesday

Breakfast: fruit compote bake; cold millet with rice milk

Lunch: Spinach Mushroom Soup; endive and chicory salad

Dinner: Honey Ginger Shrimp and Udon; Steamed Fennel Wedges;* roasted red peppers; miso kombu broth

Thursday

Breakfast: apple smoothie; mochi with sunflower butter

Lunch: Fennel Nutmeg Bisque (hot or cold); mixed greens and cold udon noodles with Miso Umeboshi Sauce

Dinner: seitan sautéed with mirin and mixed vegetables;* pinto beans;* brown rice with black sesame seeds; miso kombu broth

---

* Starred reference indicates that you should make extra for meals the next day.

Friday

Breakfast: Country Breakfast Scramble; flat bread; peaches

Lunch: Pinto Bean and Carrot Sage Ragout; brown rice salad with mixed vegetables and sesame oil

Dinner: tempeh with daikon and burdock; bulghur wheat* with pine nuts; mustard greens; miso soup with ginger and scallions

Saturday

Breakfast: stewed pears and berries; bulghur wheat (hot or cold) with rice milk

Lunch: Walnut Sage Paté on flat bread; miso soup with scallions

Dinner: seitan fried with leeks and mushrooms; steamed squash;* kidney beans;* rosa rice*

Sunday

Breakfast: millet squash porridge; mochi with sunflower butter

Lunch: New Orleans Red Beans and Rice; miso kombu broth

Dinner: Refrigerator Reincarnations (see page 87 for instructions)

---

* Starred reference indicates that you should make extra for meals the next day.

PART FOUR

Recipes

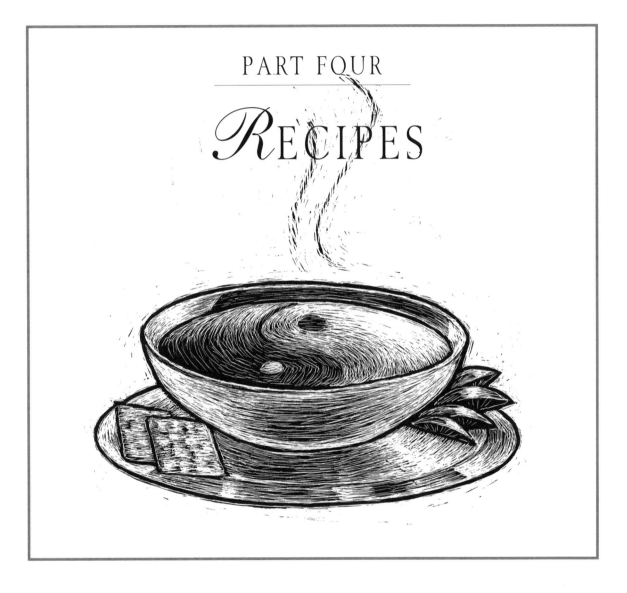

10

APPETIZERS AND
PARTY DISHES

Squash and Red Pepper Roll-Ups
Serves 6

These colorful little pinwheels make the perfect healthy party appetizer. Or try serving them whole as a tasty alternative to the traditional lunchtime sandwich.

3 cups cubed yellow squash
$^1/_4$ pound silken low-fat tofu
1 tablespoon barley malt syrup
1 tablespoon corn oil
1 medium yellow onion, minced
1 medium red pepper, diced
1 teaspoon unrefined sea salt
$^1/_2$ cup coarsely chopped cilantro
6 large whole-wheat tortillas

In a large saucepan, steam the squash just until tender. Combine with the tofu and barley malt syrup in a blender, and puree until smooth.

Heat the oil in a medium skillet. Sauté the onions, red peppers, and salt until the onions are translucent. Add the onion mixture to the squash mixture. Stir in the cilantro.

Cool the mixture well and spread evenly on the tortillas. Roll up tightly and secure with toothpicks. Chill for several hours, then slice 1 inch thick before serving.

Southwestern Avocado and Corn Dip

Makes 3 cups

This rich but healthy appetizer is a lighter version of traditional guacamole, with sweet corn and reduced-fat tofu for a fresh, unique taste. Use apple slices instead of fried tortilla chips for dipping for an even healthier snack.

1 large avocado, cubed
$1/2$ pound silken low-fat tofu
1 cup fresh corn kernels
1 medium yellow onion, finely chopped
$1/2$ cup finely chopped cilantro
$1/2$ teaspoon white pepper
1 teaspoon unrefined sea salt

Garnish
Sprigs of cilantro

Puree the avocado and tofu in a blender until smooth. Stir in the corn, onions, cilantro, white pepper, and salt.

Transfer the dip to a serving dish, and garnish with cilantro. Use as a spread on warmed whole-wheat tortillas, or serve with thin slices of crisp, chilled apples for dipping.

Broccoli and Wild Rice Pancakes

Serves 4

These unexpected treats make a wonderful first course for a special dinner or an easy, exotic appetizer.

2 cups broccoli
$1/2$ cup cooked wild rice
$1/2$ cup cooked brown rice
1 cup garbanzo flour
2 tablespoons gomashio
$1/2$ cup soy milk
1 tablespoon safflower oil

Cut the broccoli into florets. Peel the stems and slice. Using a large pot, steam in 1 inch of boiling water for 5 to 10 minutes or until tender. Puree in a blender with a little cooking water until smooth.

Combine the wild rice, brown rice, flour, and gomashio in a large mixing bowl, and mix well. Stir in the broccoli puree and soy milk.

Heat the oil in a medium skillet; drop the batter by tablespoonfuls into the skillet. Cook until browned on both sides, turning carefully.

Serve hot with Mushroom Gravy or Raisin Peach Chutney.

Walnut Sage Paté
Makes 3 cups

This tasty paté is a high-protein, vegetarian substitute for the meat version, with a nutty, rich flavor.

2 cups cooked lentils
$^1/_2$ pound silken low-fat tofu
1 tablespoon olive oil
$^1/_2$ cup fresh sage, chopped, with stems removed
1 teaspoon white pepper
1 teaspoon unrefined sea salt
$^1/_2$ cup chopped walnuts

Combine all ingredients in a blender, and puree until very smooth. Serve as a spread on bread or crackers, or as a dip with fresh vegetables.

Sprouted Hummus
Makes 5 cups

Sprouted garbanzo beans and basil add texture, extra nutrition, and an unexpected taste to this updated version of a traditional Middle Eastern favorite.

3 cups cooked garbanzo beans
$^1/_2$ cup tahini
3 cloves garlic, crushed
1 teaspoon unrefined sea salt
$^1/_4$ cup brown rice vinegar
1 cup sprouted garbanzo beans
$^1/_4$ cup chopped basil

Combine the cooked garbanzo beans, tahini, garlic, salt, and brown rice vinegar in a blender. Puree until smooth, adding water as needed to make a creamy mixture. Pour the mixture into a medium bowl.

Place the sprouted garbanzo beans in the blender and process briefly on low speed to make a thick, crumbly mixture.

Stir the sprouted garbanzo beans and basil into the hummus mixture, and chill before serving. Spread on chapati or pita, or serve as a dip with assorted raw vegetables.

Chickpea Fritters with Apple Date Chutney
Makes 12 fritters

Thick, fragrant chutney brings out the flavor of these delicately spiced finger foods—ideal as an appetizer or a side dish with dinner.

3 cups garbanzo (chickpea) flour
2 cups water
1 teaspoon unrefined sea salt
1/2 cup cauliflower in small florets
1/2 cup diced carrots
1/2 cup fresh garden peas
1/2 cup diced red onions
2 cloves garlic, minced
2 tablespoons cumin seed
Sunflower oil

Chutney:
1 cup chopped and pitted dates
1 large apple, finely chopped
1/2 cup raisins
1/2 cup honey
1/2 cup brown rice vinegar

Mix the flour, water, and salt in a medium bowl, stirring gently. Set aside.

Steam the cauliflower, carrots, peas, and onions until tender (about 10 minutes).

Combine the garlic, cumin seed, and steamed vegetables, and stir into the chickpea batter.

Preheat the oven to 250°F. Lightly coat a heavy skillet with oil and heat over medium heat. Drop the batter into the skillet by heaping tablespoons. Brown on both sides, pressing down gently with a spatula, then remove to an ovenproof platter. Keep the fritters warm in the oven until ready to serve.

To make the chutney, which may be prepared ahead of time, combine all the ingredients in a medium saucepan. Bring to a full boil, then simmer for 15 minutes until thick, stirring frequently. Serve hot or at room temperature as a dipping sauce with the fritters.

Winter Squash Triangles
Makes 12 triangles

Stuffed with a creamy sweet mixture of root vegetables and delicate spices, these flat-bread sandwiches make tasty appetizers and luscious lunch fare.

2 cups cubed butternut squash
1 cup cubed sweet potato
1 tablespoon safflower oil
$^{1}/_{2}$ cup finely chopped scallions
1 teaspoon unrefined sea salt
1 clove garlic, crushed
1 tablespoon brown rice syrup
2 teaspoons nutmeg
2 teaspoons cinnamon
$^{1}/_{2}$ cup tahini
6 whole-wheat tortillas

In a large pot, steam the squash and sweet potato over medium-high heat until tender (about 30 minutes using a regular pot). Let the squash mixture cool slightly.

While the squash is cooking, heat the oil and sauté the scallions, salt, and garlic in a medium saucepan until the scallions are translucent. Add the brown rice syrup, nutmeg, and cinnamon.

Puree the squash mixture with tahini until smooth. Combine the scallion mixture with the pureed squash mixture.

Warm the tortillas in a dry skillet, heating each side for about 1 minute. Spread $^{1}/_{2}$ cup filling on each tortilla and fold in half. Cut in half to form two triangles. Chill thoroughly or serve warm.

Garbanzo Beet Chapati

Makes 12 chapati

The distinctive flavor of garbanzo flour and the kick of cumin team up with colorful beets to make an unexpected—but delightful—variation on traditional chapati.

2½ cups garbanzo (chickpea) flour
1 teaspoon unrefined sea salt
2 tablespoons cumin seed
1 cup beet juice
1 medium yellow onion, finely chopped
Additional flour for rolling chapati

Mix the flour, salt, and cumin in a medium bowl. Slowly stir in the beet juice and onions. Turn the dough onto a wooden board covered with flour, and knead for 5 minutes to form a smooth dough, adding water or flour as needed. Let rest, covered with a damp cloth, for 15 minutes.

Preheat the oven to 200°F.

Heat a large, heavy skillet over medium-high heat. Divide the dough into 12 balls, dredge each in the remaining flour, and roll out into thin, 5-inch circles.

Cook the chapati for 1 to 2 minutes on each side, gently pressing down with a spatula to flatten (the chapati will form small brownish spots rather than turning a uniform brown color). Stack on an ovenproof plate, cover with a slightly damp cloth, and keep warm in a low oven. Serve with soups and main courses, or with spreads and dips as an appetizer.

Layered Bean Casserole
Serves 6

This deceptively simple casserole, with its unique, crunchy brown rice crust, is a perfect party meal in a dish and makes a tasty main dish of leftover beans and grains.

3 cups cooked brown rice
1 cup grated Cheddar soy cheese
1 small onion, thinly sliced
$\frac{1}{2}$ cup sliced button mushrooms
1 medium red pepper, sliced into thin rings
$\frac{1}{2}$ cup silken low-fat tofu
1 cup cooked beans (black turtle, kidney, azuki, or anasazi)
1 garlic clove, minced
1 teaspoon unrefined sea salt
1 teaspoon cumin

Preheat the oven to 375°F.

Press the cooked brown rice into a lightly oiled, medium-size glass casserole, forming a "crust" along the bottom and sides. Layer with $\frac{1}{2}$ cup soy cheese, onion, mushrooms, and red pepper.

Puree the tofu until very smooth, and combine with the beans, garlic, salt, and cumin. Spoon the mixture on top of the casserole filling, and press gently into the pan.

Bake for 30 minutes. Sprinkle the top with the remaining soy cheese and bake 5–10 minutes longer, until the vegetables are tender and the cheese is bubbly.

Poppyseed Onion Chapati

Makes 12 chapati

These savory, pancakelike concoctions are perfect with dishes and spreads that require a more hearty unleavened bread than tortillas. Best of all, they're virtually fat free.

2$^1/_2$ cups whole-wheat pastry flour
1 teaspoon unrefined sea salt
$^1/_4$ cup poppyseeds
1 medium yellow onion, finely chopped
$^1/_2$ cup water
$^1/_2$ cup soy milk
Additional flour for rolling chapati

Mix the flour, salt, poppyseeds, and onion in a large mixing bowl. Slowly stir in the water and soy milk. Turn the dough onto a wooden board coated with flour, and knead for 5 minutes to form a smooth dough, adding water and flour as needed. Let rest, covered with a damp cloth, for 15 minutes.

Preheat the oven to 200°F.

Heat a large skillet over medium-high heat. Divide the dough into 12 balls; coat each ball lightly with flour and roll out into thin, 5-inch circles.

Cook the chapatis for 1 to 2 minutes on each side until lightly browned, gently pressing down with a spatula (the chapati will form small, brown spots rather than turn a uniform brown color). Stack them on an ovenproof plate, cover with a cloth, and keep warm in the oven.

Nori Rolls (Maki Sushi)
Makes 8 rolls

These tempting vegetarian takes on the traditional fish dish are perfect party dishes with dipping sauces and garnishes. Or, for a fast, nutritious lunch, leave the rolls whole and serve with simple sauces.

8 sheets nori
3 cups cooked short-grain brown rice or Kokuko rose rice
1 cup thinly sliced vegetables (cucumber, carrot, daikon, burdock, scallions, seitan, watercress, other cooked vegetables)
1 tablespoon umeboshi plum paste
$^{1}/_{4}$ cup black or regular sesame seeds

Lay each sheet of nori flat on a bamboo sushi mat, and spread about $^{1}/_{3}$ cup rice over about three-fourths of the nori. Lay the filling lengthwise about 1 inch from the bottom edge of the nori. Dot umeboshi plum paste over the vegetables, and sprinkle with sesame seeds. Starting at the bottom of the nori sheet, roll the nori up tightly, wetting the top edge to seal the roll. Slice into 1-inch rounds with a very sharp, slightly moistened knife, and serve with dipping sauces such as Creamy Ginger Dressing, Peanut Ginger Dressing, or Miso Umeboshi Sauce.

Variations: To use a spiral rolling technique, use your hands to roll the nori from both ends until the ends meet in the middle. Turn the rolled side down, and slice with a sharp, slightly moistened knife.

Cooked seafood, including crab, shrimp, and whitefish, may also be added. Serve fish sushi with side dishes of pickled ginger, grated daikon, and wasabi and tamari for dipping.

Also try substituting cooked noodles for the rice, or use leafy leftover greens as wrappers instead of sheets of nori.

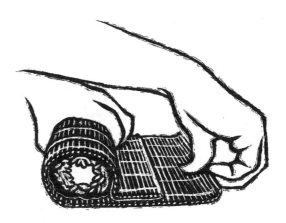

Aemono-aisho-ae

Serves 4

Although eggs are generally not used in the basic macrobiotic diet, this traditional dish, served on special occasions, takes exception to the rule.

2 cups spinach or chard
6 whole scallions
1/4 cup coarsely chopped peanuts
1/4 cup sesame seeds
1 tablespoon miso
2 eggs
2 teaspoons sunflower oil

Steam the greens and scallions until tender; cool and cut into 1/2-inch-long strips. Roast the peanuts and sesame seeds in a heavy skillet until browned, and process in a food mill or blender, adding water to form a creamy paste. Add miso, and mix with the vegetables. Beat the eggs well. Heat the oil in a large skillet and fry the eggs to make a thin, crêpelike sheet. Cool and cut into thin strips, arrange on a large platter, and cover with cooked greens.

11

SALADS

Asparagus and Yellow Pepper Toss
Serves 4 to 6

A wonderful side dish or salad to dress up any meal. Add small cubes of mozzarella-style soy cheese for an even more festive touch.

3 medium yellow peppers
1 1/2 pounds asparagus, washed well, with tough stems removed
1/4 cup brown rice vinegar
1/4 cup olive oil
2 tablespoons brown rice syrup
1 tablespoon gomashio

Garnish
1/2 red pepper, slivered

Preheat the oven to 400°F.

Cut the yellow peppers into 8 sections each and remove the stems and seeds. Place in a lightly oiled glass casserole and cook for 20 minutes, stirring frequently. Remove from the oven and cool.

While the peppers are cooking, steam the asparagus in a large saucepan until bright green and tender (5–10 minutes). Rinse with cool water and drain well.

Blend the brown rice vinegar, oil, brown rice syrup, and gomashio. Combine the asparagus, peppers, and dressing, and toss to coat well. Garnish with slivers of red peppers and serve at room temperature.

Crunchy Quinoa Salad
Serves 6

This super-healthy salad combines the delicate, nutty flavor of high-protein quinoa with nutritious seaweed and crunchy vegetables.

1 cup quinoa
2 cups water
$^1/_2$ cup diced carrots
2 bunches scallions, sliced
$^1/_2$ cup diced celery
$^1/_2$ cup chopped almonds
$^1/_2$ cup lightly soaked arame
$^1/_4$ cup tamari
$^1/_4$ cup tahini
$^1/_4$ cup mirin
1 tablespoon gomashio

Toast the quinoa in a medium pot for 2 to 3 minutes, or until the grains begin to brown. Add the water and bring to a boil; cover and simmer 15 minutes, then remove from the heat and let stand 10 minutes.

While the quinoa is cooking, combine the carrots, scallions, celery, almonds, and arame in a large mixing bowl.

In a separate, smaller bowl, make the dressing by combining the tamari, tahini, mirin, and gomashio. Stir the dressing into the vegetable mixture.

Stir the quinoa into the vegetable and dressing mixture, and chill slightly before serving.

Bitter Greens with Raspberry Poppyseed Vinaigrette
Serves 4

Served with a fruity vinaigrette, the slightly bitter flavor of mixed field greens is a fresh, lively start for any meal.

2 medium Belgian endives
1 medium head radicchio
$^1/_2$ cup curly chicory
$^1/_2$ cup arugula
$^1/_2$ cup red oak leaf lettuce
$^1/_2$ cup mustard greens
$^1/_2$ cup Raspberry Poppyseed Vinaigrette (page 179)

Thoroughly wash all the lettuce. Cut the endive into $^1/_4$-inch slices, and tear other lettuces into bite-size pieces.

Toss the salad in a large, decorative bowl with the dressing. Garnish with pine nuts if desired, and serve immediately.

Wild Side Salad
Serves 4

A combination of wild rice, nuts, shiitake mushrooms, and a zesty sauce makes this crunchy, nutty salad an unforgettable first-course or party dish.

2 teaspoons light sesame oil
1 cup sliced shiitake mushrooms
1 cup wild rice
1 cup brown rice
$^1/_4$ cup chopped almonds
$^1/_4$ cup chopped pecans
$^1/_4$ cup lightly soaked hijiki
1 bunch scallions, sliced, with green tops
$^1/_2$ cup Miso Umeboshi Sauce (page 177)

Heat the oil in a medium saucepan, and sauté the shiitake until limp.

Combine all the ingredients in a large mixing bowl, and toss well to coat with the dressing. Chill to allow the flavors to mix before serving.

Mixed Grains with Seitan and Pumpkin Seeds
Serves 6 to 8

A wonderful way to use leftover rice and other grains, this dish is savory and satisfying served either hot or cold. For a hearty, hot side dish, use a little more gravy.

1 tablespoon almond oil
1 cup cubed seitan
1 bunch scallions, sliced (including greens)
$^1/_2$ cup sliced button or shiitake mushrooms
$^1/_2$ cup diced carrots
$^1/_4$ cup sake
1 tablespoon gomashio
$^1/_2$ cup arame
$^1/_2$ to 1 cup Mushroom Gravy (page 176)
$^1/_2$ cup pumpkin seeds
2 cups cooked brown rice, quinoa, buckwheat, millet, or other grains

Heat the oil in a medium skillet. Add the seitan, scallions, mushrooms, carrots, and gomashio, and sauté on medium heat, adding sake as needed to prevent sticking, until the carrots are tender.

Combine the vegetable mixture, arame, Mushroom Gravy, pumpkin seeds, and grains in a medium mixing bowl. Chill slightly. Serve as a salad over a bed of field greens, or serve warm as a side dish.

Festive Pepper Salad
Serves 4 to 6

A colorful combination of sweet red peppers and bitter greens, with crunchy, nutritious sprouts and a fresh dressing, this dish lives up to its name.

2 teaspoons olive oil
$^1/_2$ cup sliced daikon
2 medium red peppers, cut into $^1/_4$-inch slices
2 Belgian endive, cut into rounds
$^1/_2$ cup cooked corn
$^1/_2$ cup mung bean sprouts
1 cup Apple Basil Vinaigrette (page 180)

Heat the oil in a medium skillet, and sauté the daikon until tender. Let cool.

Combine all the ingredients in a medium bowl, and toss with the dressing until well coated. Chill before serving to allow the flavor to blend.

Corn and Buckwheat Crunch
Serves 4

This appetizer-style salad, with its combination of hearty, chewy grains and crunchy, sweet corn, is a wonderful way to use leftover buckwheat. Other grains can be substituted or added in place of a portion of the buckwheat.

1½ cups cooked buckwheat
1 bunch scallions, thinly sliced (including green tops)
1 cup cooked corn kernels
½ cup grated red cabbage
1 tablespoon light sesame oil
2 tablespoons tamari
1 tablespoon gomashio
½ cup lightly soaked hijiki

Combine the buckwheat and vegetables in a medium bowl, and add the oil, tamari, gomashio, and hijiki. Stir until well mixed, and chill before serving to let the flavors blend.

Watercress Beets with Walnuts
Serves 4 to 6

Sweet beets and peppery watercress team up for a tangy, sweet taste treat in this unique, low-fat salad.

2 cups cooked beets, julienned
1 large bunch watercress, rinsed well and chopped, with stems removed
½ cup walnuts
¼ cup brown rice syrup
2 tablespoons brown rice vinegar
2 tablespoons mirin
1 tablespoon tahini
1 tablespoon gomashio

Combine the beets, watercress, and walnuts in a large bowl.
    Mix the remaining ingredients until smooth, and toss with the beets. Serve chilled.

Sprout Salad
Serves 4

This quick-and-easy, crunchy salad makes a fresh, low-fat start to any meal.

1 cup sprouted azuki, mung or garbanzo beans
1 cup sprouted sunflower seeds
1 cup radish or alfalfa sprouts
¹/₄ cup tahini
¹/₄ cup apple juice
2 tablespoons brown rice vinegar
2 tablespoons mellow white miso
1 teaspoon gomashio
¹/₄ cup slivered carrots
¹/₄ cup grated daikon

Combine the sprouts in a medium bowl. In a small bowl, mix the tahini, apple juice, brown rice vinegar, miso, and gomashio until smooth. Toss with the sprouts, garnish with carrots and daikon, and serve as a salad or side dish.

Chilled Asparagus with Ginger Dressing
Serves 4

Tender stalks of bright green asparagus make a delicious debut with the Oriental flavors of sea vegetables and ginger.

2 cups asparagus, tough stems removed
1 cup shredded red cabbage
¹/₂ pound extra-firm tofu, cut in ¹/₂-inch cubes
1 tablespoon sesame oil
1 tablespoon tamari
¹/₂ cup lightly soaked hijiki, arame, or sliced wakame
1 cup Creamy Ginger Dressing (page 178)

Steam the asparagus and cabbage for 5 minutes, or just until tender. Rinse with cold water immediately after cooking.

While the vegetables are steaming, sauté the tofu in the oil and tamari until lightly browned.

Combine the tofu and sea vegetables in a medium mixing bowl. Add the asparagus, cabbage, and dressing, and mix gently. Chill before serving to allow the flavors to blend.

Seven-Bean Salad with Creamy Ginger Dressing
Serves 4

This fast and easy, super-nutritious lunch is a perfect way to use leftover beans. Mix as many as you'd like, and substitute some sprouted beans for cooked beans.

2 cups any combination cooked or sprouted legumes (azukis, black beans, mung beans, lentils, navy beans, pinto beans, peas)
$^1/_2$ cup finely chopped scallions, including green tops
$^1/_2$ cup grated carrots
$^1/_2$ cup lightly soaked arame
$^3/_4$ cup Creamy Ginger Dressing (page 178)

Combine all the ingredients in a large mixing bowl and toss well to coat with the dressing. Chill to allow the flavors to mix before serving.

Egg-Less Salad
Makes 2 cups

This low-fat (1.5 grams compared with the 18 grams in regular egg salad) alternative to egg salad can be made with silken tofu for a creamier texture, or with firm tofu for a more traditional taste.

2 teaspoons brown rice vinegar
1 tablespoon brown rice syrup
1 tablespoon brown mustard
1 teaspoon turmeric
1 teaspoon unrefined sea salt
1 teaspoon white pepper
1 pound low-fat tofu (silken or firm, or $^1/_2$ pound of each)
$^1/_2$ cup diced celery
$^1/_4$ cup thinly sliced scallions

Combine the brown rice vinegar, brown rice syrup, mustard, turmeric, salt, and white pepper in a small bowl, and mix well.

Crumble the tofu into a mixing bowl. Add the vinegar mixture, and gently stir in the celery and scallions.

Refrigerate for several hours or overnight to let the flavors blend. Serve at room temperature in a pita pocket with a handful of sprouts.

Brown Rice Salad with Sesame Ginger Sauce
Serves 6 to 8

This quick, savory salad, with a multitude of contrasts in flavors and textures, is hearty enough for a meal by itself.

1 tablespoon olive oil
1 cup cubed seitan
$^1/_2$ cup chopped yellow onions
$^1/_2$ cup diced red peppers
$^1/_2$ cup sliced shiitake mushrooms
$^1/_4$ cup thinly sliced burdock root
1 cup sliced bok choy (greens and stalks)
2 cups cooked brown rice
$^1/_4$ cup sprouted azuki beans
$^1/_4$ cup sprouted lentils
$^1/_2$ cup lightly soaked hijiki

Dressing
$^3/_4$ cup tahini
$^1/_2$ cup toasted sesame oil
2 tablespoons barley malt syrup
1 tablespoon tamari
$^1/_4$ cup black sesame seeds
2 teaspoons freshly grated ginger
1 clove garlic, finely minced

Heat the oil in a medium skillet. Add the seitan, onions, peppers, mushrooms, and burdock. Sauté until the onions are translucent. Add the bok choy, and sauté 5 minutes longer. Remove from heat and cool.

Combine the rice with the seitan mixture in a large mixing bowl. Add the azuki sprouts, lentil sprouts, and hijiki.

To make the dressing, mix the tahini, sesame oil, barley malt syrup, and tamari in a small bowl, adding water as needed. Add the sesame seeds, ginger, and garlic. Stir into the rice mixture, and chill before serving.

Sunny Tofu Salad
Makes 6 to 8 servings

A luscious, low-fat sandwich spread with a nutty flavor that blends crunchy vegetables with creamy tofu.

$^1/_2$ pound firm low-fat tofu
1 (10-ounce) package silken tofu
$^1/_2$ cup miso
$^1/_4$ cup sunflower butter
$^1/_2$ cup finely chopped scallions
$^1/_2$ cup finely chopped red peppers
$^1/_2$ cup finely chopped parsley
1 teaspoon black pepper
1 tablespoon gomashio
$^1/_4$ cup sprouted sunflower seeds
$^1/_4$ cup sprouted mung beans

Puree the tofu, miso, and sunflower butter in a blender until smooth.

Combine the scallions, red peppers, parsley, black pepper, gomashio, sunflower seeds, and mung beans in a medium bowl, and stir in the tofu mixture.

Spread the mixture on tortillas, unleavened bread, or Poppyseed Onion Chapati.

Belgian Endive and Burdock
Serves 4

East meets West in this lively combination of crunchy bitter greens, colorful carrots and traditional Japanese root vegetables. Serve with Miso Umeboshi Sauce for an Oriental flavor, or with Apple Basil Vinaigrette for a more Western flair.

1 (5-inch-long) section daikon root, sliced into half moons
1 (10-inch-long) section burdock root, thinly sliced on the diagonal
4 heads Belgian endive
2 medium carrots, sliced on the diagonal
$^1/_2$ cup mung or lentil sprouts
1 cup Miso Umeboshi Sauce (page 177) or Apple Basil Vinaigrette (page 180)

Lightly steam the daikon and burdock in $^1/_2$ inch boiling water, in a medium saucepan, just until tender. Rinse with cold water to cool and to stop the cooking, and drain thoroughly.

Slice the Belgian endive into rounds, and combine with the daikon, burdock, carrots, and mung or lentil sprouts in a medium mixing bowl. Toss with the dressing, and chill before serving to allow the flavors to blend.

12

SOUPS AND STEWS

Fennel Nutmeg Bisque
Serves 4

This smooth, creamy soup, with the unexpected flavor of anise, makes a satisfying lunch, served with hot sourdough bread, or an elegant start to a special dinner.

1 tablespoon olive oil
1 medium yellow onion, chopped
2 cloves garlic, crushed
1 teaspoon unrefined sea salt
2 tablespoons whole-wheat flour
4 cups Light Vegetable Stock (page 139)
3 cups chopped fennel bulb
1 teaspoon white pepper
1 to 2 teaspoons nutmeg
1/4 cup chopped basil

Heat the oil in a large pot and sauté the onions and salt until the onions are translucent. Add the flour and cook 2 to 3 minutes, stirring constantly. Slowly add the stock and stir until smooth.

Stir in the fennel, and bring to a boil. Cook over medium heat until the fennel is tender (about 15 minutes).

Add the white pepper and nutmeg, and puree the soup in a blender until very smooth. Return to the pot, stir in the basil, and simmer for 5 minutes to let the flavors blend.

Pinto Bean and Carrot Sage Ragout
Serves 4 to 6

This rich stew is a wonderful way to sneak beans into your daily diet. Mung beans may be substituted for pintos for a variation on flavors.

1 tablepoon olive oil
1 leek, sliced (including green top)
6 carrots, chopped
1 teaspoon unrefined sea salt
3 cups Rich Vegetable Stock (see the variation of Light Vegetable Stock, page 139)
1 cup soaked pinto beans
1 cup soy milk
$1/4$ cup finely chopped fresh sage

Heat the oil in a large pot and sauté the leeks, carrots, and salt until the vegetables are tender.

Add the stock and pinto beans, and bring to a boil. Lower the heat and simmer 1 to $1^1/2$ hours, or until the beans are tender.

Add the soy milk and sage, and simmer 5 minutes longer. Serve with hearty sourdough bread.

Note: For faster preparation, cooked pinto beans may be substituted for uncooked pinto beans. To prepare with precooked beans, sauté the vegetables, then add the stock and cooked beans and heat through. Add the soy milk and sage, and simmer 5 minutes longer.

Red Lentil Soup with Arame
Serves 4 to 6

This colorful twist on the standard brown lentil soup is a simple dinner dish and makes wonderful next-day leftover lunches.

2 teaspoons olive oil
1 medium onion, diced
1 clove garlic, minced
3 carrots, chopped
$^1/_2$ teaspoon unrefined sea salt
2 tablespoons each fresh thyme, basil, sage, and rosemary
4 cups Rich Vegetable Stock (see the variation of Light Vegetable Stock, page 139)
$^1/_2$ teaspoon black pepper
1 cup red lentils
$^1/_4$ cup tamari
$^1/_2$ cup lightly soaked arame
$^1/_4$ cup sake

Heat the oil in a large pot and sauté the onions, garlic, carrots, and salt until the onions are translucent.

Add the herbs, stock, black pepper, and lentils, and bring to a boil. Lower the heat and simmer 30 minutes.

Add the tamari and arame, and cook for 15 minutes longer. Stir in the sake and serve.

Black Bean Soup with Roasted Red Peppers

Serves 4 to 6

Serve this hearty soup with white or brown basmati rice—its delicate taste complements the smoky flavors of the beans and roasted peppers.

2 whole red peppers
1 tablespoon olive oil
1 medium white onion, chopped
1 clove garlic, minced
2 cups cooked black beans
3 cups Rich Vegetable Stock (see the variation of Light Vegetable Stock, page 139)
1 bunch cilantro, coarsely chopped
2 teaspoons cumin

To roast the red peppers, place them on a baking sheet in a 400°F. oven for 30 minutes, turning several times until evenly charred on all sides. Wrap the peppers in a damp towel to cool; then peel off the charred skin, remove the stems and seeds, and cut into 1/2-inch strips.

Heat the oil in a large saucepan. Add the onions and garlic, and sauté over medium heat until the onions are translucent.

Add the beans and stock, and simmer for 10 minutes. Add the cilantro, cumin, and red peppers. Simmer 5 more minutes, and serve with basmati rice and a side dish of leafy green vegetables.

Borscht with Beans
Serves 4 to 6

This creative take on the traditional Russian beet soup adds pinto beans for extra nutrition and additional texture.

2 tablespoons safflower oil
1 cup grated green cabbage
6 large beets, grated
1 medium yellow onion, diced
$^1/_4$ cup brown rice syrup
$^1/_2$ cup brown rice vinegar
4 cups Light Vegetable Stock (page 139)
1 cup cooked pinto beans
$^1/_2$ pound silken low-fat tofu
2 tablespoons brown rice vinegar
1 tablespoon caraway seeds

Heat the oil in a large pot. Sauté the cabbage, beets, and onions until the beets are tender (about 5–10 minutes). Stir in the brown rice syrup and brown rice vinegar, and cook 5 minutes longer.

Add the stock, then cover the pot and simmer for 20 minutes. Pour the soup into a blender and puree until smooth. Return to the pot and stir in the beans.

Puree the tofu and 2 tablespoons brown rice vinegar until very smooth. Serve each portion of borscht hot, with a dollop of the pureed tofu and a sprinkle of caraway seeds.

Carrot Coconut Bisque with Cilantro
Serves 4

This rich soup combines the fresh, sweet flavor of carrots with subtle undertones of cilantro.

3 cups chopped carrots
1 small yellow onion, finely chopped
2 cups coconut milk (a mixture of 1 cup coconut milk and 1 cup light soy milk may be used)
1 teaspoon nutmeg
$^1/_2$ teaspoon white pepper
1 teaspoon unrefined sea salt
$^1/_2$ cup chopped cilantro

Garnish
Fresh cilantro sprigs

Place the carrots in a large soup pot with just enough water to cover. Cook covered over medium heat until tender. Add the onions and cook 5 minutes longer.

Add the coconut milk (or coconut and soy milk), nutmeg, pepper, and salt, and puree in a blender until very smooth.

Return the mixture to the pot, and stir in the cilantro. Cook over low heat just until warmed through (do not overcook or the coconut milk will lose its delicate flavor). Garnish with fresh sprigs of cilantro, and serve in small bowls with braised greens and basmati rice on the side.

Cream of Celery Soup
Serves 4 to 6

This creamy, delicate soup can be served either hot or cold. Try sprinkling the top with a little dill or poppyseeds for garnish.

1 tablespoon olive oil
2 heads celery, chopped
1 small yellow onion, chopped
$1/2$ teaspoon unrefined sea salt
1 teaspoon celery seed
$1/2$ teaspoon white pepper
1 tablespoon flour
2 cups Light Vegetable Stock (page 139)
$1/2$ pound silken low-fat tofu
1 cup soy milk

Heat the oil in a large pot and sauté the celery, onions, and salt until the celery is tender.

Add the celery seed, white pepper, and flour, and stir until the vegetables are well coated. Cook slowly over medium heat for 2 minutes, stirring constantly. Slowly stir in the stock and cook 5 minutes longer.

Puree the tofu and soy milk with the celery mixture until very smooth. Return the mixture to the pot, heat through and serve hot, or chill for several hours.

Wild Mushroom and Barley Stew
Serves 6 to 8

Hearty seitan and barley, balanced with the delicate smoky flavor of wild mushrooms, combine to make a rich and satisfying stew.

2 tablespoons corn oil
¼ cup each thinly sliced shiitake, porcini, chanterelle, and morel
   mushrooms
½ cup sliced button mushrooms
1 medium leek, sliced (including green top)
1 teaspoon unrefined sea salt
2 tablespoons whole-wheat flour
1 cup soy milk
2 cups Rich Vegetable Stock (see the variation of Light Vegetable Stock,
   page 139)
1 cup cubed seitan
1 cup cooked barley
¼ cup finely chopped fresh rosemary

Heat the oil in a medium saucepan, and add the mushrooms, leeks, and salt. Sauté until the mushrooms are soft and the leeks are translucent.

Add the flour and stir until the vegetables are coated. Cook over medium-low heat for 2 minutes, stirring constantly. Slowly stir in the soy milk and stock. Cook for 2 minutes longer, or until thick and bubbly.

Add the seitan and barley to the soup stock, and simmer until the seitan is heated through (5 to 7 minutes), stirring frequently. Just before serving, stir in the rosemary and sprinkle the top with thin slices of mushrooms.

Creamy Watercress Soup
Serves 4

Pungent, peppery watercress gives this soup a special kick. Serve chilled for a refreshing lunch treat on a hot summer day.

2 teaspoons safflower oil
1 medium yellow onion, finely diced
1 teaspoon unrefined sea salt
1 teaspoon black pepper
1 tablespoon flour
2 cups Light Vegetable Stock (page 139)
3 bunches watercress, chopped, with stems removed
1 cup soy milk
¼ cup sake

Heat the oil in a medium pot. Sauté the onions, salt, and black pepper until the onions are translucent.

Stir in the flour and cook for 1 to 2 minutes, stirring constantly. Slowly whisk in the stock and beat until creamy and thickened.

Add the watercress and cook for about 10 minutes. Stir in the soy milk, then pour the mixture into a blender and puree quickly (about 3–5 seconds), leaving large pieces of watercress. Stir in the sake and serve.

Zucchini Bisque
Serves 4 to 6

This creamy concoction uses coconut milk for a distinctive flavor. Serve it on special occasions, or use light soy milk instead of coconut milk for still-scrumptious, low-fat fare.

4 medium zucchini, cubed
1 medium yellow onion, chopped
1 teaspoon white pepper
1 teaspoon unrefined sea salt
2 cups coconut milk (a mixture of half coconut milk and half light soy milk may be used)
1 small carrot, coarsely grated

Steam the zucchini and onions in a large soup pot until tender (5–10 minutes).

Puree the zucchini mixture with the white pepper, salt, and coconut milk. Return the mixture to the saucepan; add the grated carrot and heat through (don't overcook—the delicate flavor of coconut milk is destroyed by heat).

Rosemary Winter Squash Stew
Serves 6

This rich-tasting soup with delicate undertones of rosemary and sage is a perfect midday meal on blustery winter days.

4 cups cubed butternut or acorn squash
1 tablespoon corn oil
1 small yellow onion, chopped
2 tablespoons whole-wheat flour
1 cup Light Vegetable Stock (page 139)
1 cup soy milk
$^{1}/_{2}$ cup mellow white miso
$^{1}/_{2}$ cup cubed low-fat firm tofu
$^{1}/_{4}$ cup chopped fresh rosemary
$^{1}/_{4}$ cup chopped fresh sage
1 teaspoon black pepper

Steam the squash in a large soup pot with a tight-fitting lid until tender (about 10 minutes).

Heat the oil in a medium saucepan. Add the onion and sauté until translucent. Stir in the flour and cook for 2 minutes, stirring constantly.

Lower the heat and slowly stir in the stock and soy milk. Heat until thick and bubbly. Add the cooked squash, miso, and tofu. Pour the mixture into a blender and puree until very smooth.

Return the pureed mixture to the pan, and stir in the rosemary, sage, and black pepper.

Hot and Sour Soup

Serves 4 to 6

This vegan version of the Chinese favorite uses firm tofu and traditional macro stock. Leftover grains or noodles can be added for variety.

2 teaspoons light sesame oil
1 medium yellow onion, chopped
1/4 cup finely grated ginger
2 medium carrots, cut into matchsticks
1 cup thinly sliced shiitake mushrooms
1/2 teaspoon unrefined sea salt
1/2 pound firm low-fat tofu, cubed
1/2 teaspoon white pepper
3 cups Kombu Dashi Stock (page 139)
1/2 cup lightly soaked arame
1/2 cup brown rice vinegar
2 tablespoons honey
1 tablespoon gomashio

Heat the oil in a large pot and sauté the onions, ginger, carrots, mushrooms, and salt until the onions are translucent. Add the tofu and white pepper, and cook for 3 to 5 minutes longer over medium-high heat.

Stir in the stock, arame, brown rice vinegar, and honey, and let the mixture simmer for 5 minutes longer.

Add the gomashio and serve immediately.

Spinach Mushroom Soup

Serves 4 to 6

This creamy, low-fat soup uses the classic combination of mushroom and spinach. Serve with hearty dark sourdough bread and Bitter Greens Salad with Raspberry Poppyseed Vinaigrette for a complete meal.

1 tablespoon olive oil
1 medium leek, chopped
2 cups chopped button mushrooms
1 teaspoon unrefined sea salt
1 teaspoon white pepper
2 tablespoons flour
2 cups Light Vegetable Stock (page 139)
1 cup soy milk
1 (10-ounce) package silken low-fat tofu
1 pound spinach, washed and chopped, with stems removed

In a large soup pot, heat the oil over medium heat. Sauté the leeks, mushrooms, salt, and pepper until the leeks are translucent.

Add the flour and stir until the vegetables are coated. Cook 2 minutes longer, stirring constantly. Whisk in the stock, and cook over medium heat until the mixture begins to thicken; then slowly add the soy milk.

Combine one-half of the leek mixture with the tofu in a food processor, and puree until very smooth. Return to the pot with the remaining soup.

Stir in the spinach. Cook over medium heat until the spinach wilts but is still bright green. Serve immediately.

Yin Yang Swirl
Serves 6

The presentation of this perfectly balanced soup (the yin comes from the white corn, the yang from the carrots) is as appealing and unique as its creamy combination of subtle flavors.

2 cups chopped carrots
2 cups soy milk
1/2 teaspoon nutmeg
1 teaspoon white pepper
2 tablespoons brown rice syrup
1/2 teaspoon unrefined sea salt
3 cups white corn kernels
1 (10-ounce) package silken low-fat tofu

Garnish
Parsley sprigs

To make the carrot soup, steam the carrots over medium-high heat in a medium saucepan until tender. Drain well. Add 1 1/2 cups soy milk, nutmeg, white pepper, brown rice syrup, and salt to the carrots. Puree in a blender until very smooth and return to the saucepan to heat through.

To make the corn soup, puree the corn kernels with the tofu and the remaining 1/2 cup soy milk. Pour into a medium saucepan and heat through.

To serve, pour both soups into a large serving bowl simultaneously. Drag a butter knife or chopstick through to create a "Yin Yang" swirl (see illustration on page 105). Garnish with a sprig of parsley.

Summer Squash Soup with Pepitas

Serves 4 to 6

This creamy yet delicate and refreshing summer soup makes a light meal in itself, served with a crisp salad and Garbanzo Beet Chapati.

4 medium yellow summer squash, cubed
1 tablespoon safflower oil
1 medium yellow onion, diced
$^1/_2$ teaspoon unrefined sea salt
1 teaspoon coarse black pepper
2 tablespoons whole-wheat flour
1 cup Light Vegetable Stock (page 139)
$^1/_2$ cup soy milk
1 (10-ounce) package silken tofu
$^1/_2$ cup pepitas

Steam the squash in large pot for 5 to 10 minutes, or just until tender.

While the squash is cooking, heat the oil in a medium saucepan. Add the onions, salt, and pepper, and sauté until the onions are translucent. Stir in the flour; lower the heat and cook slowly for 1 to 2 minutes, stirring constantly. Slowly stir in the stock and soy milk. Continue stirring over low heat until the mixture thickens.

Combine the tofu and squash in a blender, and puree on high speed until smooth. Return the mixture to the pot, and stir in the stock mixture. Heat through, and stir in pepitas just before serving.

Kombu Dashi Stock

Makes 6 cups

The nutty, rich flavor of kombu makes this traditional stock a must for macro kitchens. Use as a base for miso soups or simple noodle dishes.

6 cups water
2 (5-inch) strips kombu
$1/2$ cup dried shiitake mushrooms
$1/4$ cup bonito flakes or shaved bonito

Combine all the ingredients in a large, heavy pot and simmer uncovered over medium heat for about 20 minutes. Remove the kombu and simmer 5 minutes longer. Strain and store in a covered glass container.

Light Vegetable Stock

Makes 6 to 8 cups

This indispensable, delicately flavored broth is the versatile beginning for many a macro meal.

2 tablespoons sunflower oil
4 cups coarsely chopped vegetables (parsley, carrots, onions, celery tops, turnips, and so on)
1 teaspoon unrefined sea salt
2 quarts water
3 bay leaves
1 teaspoon celery seed

Heat the oil in a large, heavy pot. Sauté the vegetables, with the salt, for about 10 minutes, or until tender. Add the water; bring to a boil, then lower the heat and simmer for 1 to 2 hours. Strain well.

Variation: To make Rich Vegetable Stock, follow the directions above, but add 1 teaspoon black pepper and two 5-inch strips of kombu during cooking. After cooking for 1 to 2 hours, boil uncovered until reduced by about 20 percent. Remove from the heat, strain, and add 2 tablespoons red miso and 3 tablespoons nutritional yeast after stock is reduced. Up to $1/2$ cup red wine or sake may also be added after cooking, and fish bones may be used during cooking if desired.

13

MEATLESS MAIN DISHES AND FISH

Seitan and Broccoli in Ginger Garlic Sauce
Serves 4 to 6

Crisp green broccoli and a pungent sauce are the perfect complements to the hearty taste of seitan.

1 pound seitan
1 large head broccoli
1 tablespoon corn oil
$^1/_2$ cup sliced shiitake mushrooms
$^1/_4$ cup sake
1 cup Ginger Garlic Sauce (page 181)
1 tablespoon black sesame seeds

Slice the seitan $^1/_4$ inch thick into strips about $^1/_2$ inch wide and 2 inches long. After removing the tough lower stems of the broccoli, cut it lengthwise into slender pieces, leaving the tops attached to stems.

In a medium saucepan, heat the oil and sauté the mushrooms until limp. Add the seitan, broccoli, and sake, and cook over medium heat until the broccoli is tender (about 5–10 minutes).

Add the Ginger Garlic Sauce to the pan and warm through. Stir in the sesame seeds, and serve over basmati rice or noodles.

Mixed-Bean Polenta

Serves 8

A super-nutritious, easy-to-make meal in a dish with a distinct combination of colors and flavors.

2¹/₂ cups water
1 cup polenta or cornmeal
2 tablespoons sunflower oil
1 tablespoon corn oil
¹/₂ cup diced onions
¹/₂ cup sliced mushrooms
2 tablespoons flour
¹/₂ cup Light Vegetable Stock (page 139)
¹/₂ cup carrot juice
1 teaspoon cumin
1 bunch cilantro, chopped
1 cup diced red pepper
1 cup yellow corn
2 cups cooked beans (pinto, black turtle, anasazi, kidney, or other combination)

Preheat the oven to 375°F.

Bring the water to a boil and slowly whisk in the polenta or cornmeal. Cook over medium heat for 5 to 10 minutes, stirring frequently. Let the mixture cool; then press into the bottom of a large glass casserole coated with the sunflower oil.

Heat the corn oil in a medium saucepan and sauté the onions and mushrooms. Add the flour and stir until the vegetables are well coated. Cook for 1 to 2 minutes, stirring constantly.

Slowly add the stock, carrot juice, and cumin. Cook 2–3 minutes longer, until thick and bubbly. Stir in the cilantro, red pepper, corn, and beans, and heat through.

Pour the vegetable mixture into the crust and bake for 20 minutes.

Tempeh and Celery Hearts
with Mustard Tahini Sauce
Serves 4

*Tangy mustard and creamy tahini pair up in this unexpected combination of
flavors. Perfect for a hearty but fresh-tasting dinner dish.*

1 tablespoon olive oil
1 small white onion, chopped
1 cup sliced mushrooms
1 cup diagonally sliced celery hearts
$^1/_2$ teaspoon unrefined sea salt
1 tablespoon whole-wheat flour
$^1/_2$ cup water
$^1/_2$ cup sake
2 tablespoons brown mustard
2 (8-ounce) packages tempeh, crumbled
2 tablespoons tahini

Heat the oil in a large saucepan. Sauté the onions, mushrooms, celery, and salt
until the celery is tender.

Add the flour and stir until all ingredients are well coated. Cook for 1 to
2 minutes, stirring constantly. Slowly stir in the water, sake, and mustard. Add
the tempeh and cook through (about 10 minutes). Stir in the tahini just before
serving.

Seitan with Capers and Shallots
Serves 4

The classic combination of capers and shallots adds a new twist to this macro meat substitute.

1 tablespoon safflower oil
1 pound seitan, cut into 1/4-inch-thick slices (about 2 inches wide and
    3 inches long)
1 clove garlic, minced
3 shallots, finely chopped
1 cup thinly sliced mushrooms
1/4 cup capers
1/4 cup sake

Heat the oil in a medium skillet. Add the seitan, garlic, shallots, and mushrooms, and sauté over medium heat until the mushrooms are limp and the seitan is browned (about 10 minutes).

Add the capers and sake, and heat through. Serve with basmati rice and a mixed bitter-greens salad.

Almost Instant Noodles
Serves 4

This quick, low-fat noodle dish makes an easy, nutritous, and tasty dinner.

8 ounces whole-grain noodles (elbows, spirals, shells, etc.)
2 teaspoons olive oil
1 yellow onion, coarsely chopped
2 carrots, sliced on the diagonal
1 small red pepper, coarsely chopped
1 pound low-fat firm tofu
1 cup spinach, chopped
1 teaspoon unrefined sea salt
1/2 teaspoon black pepper
Dried or fresh herbs, wakame, ginger, tamari, tahini, miso (optional)

Add the noodles and olive oil to 2 quarts hot water. As the water begins to boil, add the onions, carrots, and red pepper. When the noodles are almost done (about 7 minutes), add the tofu, spinach, salt, black pepper, and any of the optional ingredients, and continue cooking until the noodles are tender.

Baked Tofu, Shallots, and Wild Mushrooms
Serves 4

Baking instead of frying makes this exotic dish a low-fat treat. Serve it to your friends who think tofu can only be bland.

1 tablespoon safflower oil
1 pound low-fat tofu, cut into 1/4-inch-thick slices
4 medium shallots, thinly sliced
1/2 pound sliced mushrooms (use a combination of chanterelles, morels, porcini, shiitake, or button mushrooms)
1 teaspoon white pepper
1 clove garlic, minced
1/4 cup finely chopped fresh basil
1/4 cup Light Vegetable Stock (page 139)
1/2 cup sake
2 tablespoons brown rice syrup
2 tablespoons tamari
1 tablespoon arrowroot

Preheat the oven to 375°F.

Coat the bottom of a glass casserole with the oil. Layer the tofu, shallots, and mushrooms in the casserole, and sprinkle with white pepper, garlic, and basil.

Combine the stock, sake, brown rice syrup, tamari, and arrowroot in a small mixing bowl. Pour over the tofu mixture.

Cover the casserole loosely with foil and bake for about 20 minutes, basting the tofu with the marinade during cooking. This casserole can be prepared ahead of time and stored in the refrigerator overnight before cooking.

Roasted Pepper Casserole
with Cilantro Millet Custard
Serves 6

This satisfying meal-in-a-dish combines a creamy millet custard with the Southwestern flavor of peppers and cilantro. Perfect for parties and as a hearty dinner meal with Crunchy Skillet Cornbread.

8 Anaheim chile peppers
1 tablespoon corn oil
2 cups cooked millet
1^1/$_2$ cups grated Cheddar-style soy cheese
^{1}/$_2$ cup soy milk
^{1}/$_2$ cup chopped red pepper
^{1}/$_2$ cup fresh corn kernels
^{1}/$_2$ cup finely chopped cilantro
1 tablespoon ground cumin

Roast the peppers on a baking sheet in a 400°F oven for 30 minutes, turning several times until evenly charred on all sides. Wrap the peppers in a damp towel to cool; then peel off the charred skin and remove the stems and seeds. (Peppers can be roasted ahead of time and stored, covered, in the refrigerator.) Reduce the oven temperature to 350°F.

Coat the bottom of a large glass casserole with the corn oil. Cut the peppers in quarters and arrange on the bottom of the casserole.

Combine the millet, 1 cup soy cheese, soy milk, red pepper, corn, cilantro, and cumin in a medium saucepan. Heat until the cheese melts and the custard becomes thick and creamy.

Spread the millet mixture on top of the peppers, and sprinkle with the remaining soy cheese. Bake for 20 minutes. Let cool slightly to set before serving.

Tempeh and Burdock with Red Pepper Puree
Serves 4

The sweet, smoky flavor of roasted red peppers gives traditional macrobiotic ingredients an exotic twist in this quick and easy dish.

2 (8-ounce) packages tempeh
1 teaspoon light sesame oil
2 teaspoons toasted sesame oil
1 medium burdock root, slivered
1 cup thinly sliced shiitake mushrooms
1 tablespoon gomashio
$^1/_2$ cup mirin or sake
1 to 2 cups Red Pepper Puree (page 178)

Cut the tempeh block into quarters, then cut each quarter diagonally to form triangles. Slice each triangle in half lengthwise to make a total of 32 thin triangles.

Heat the oils in a medium skillet. Add the tempeh, burdock, mushrooms, and gomashio, and sauté over medium heat until the burdock is very tender and the tempeh is thoroughly cooked (about 10 minutes). Add the mirin or sake as needed during cooking to prevent sticking.

Remove the mixture from the pan and pour heated Red Pepper Puree over the tempeh. Serve with wild rice or quinoa and lightly steamed, leafy greens.

Wild Mushroom Polenta

Serves 4 to 6

This creamy casserole combines the fresh, green taste of spinach with flavorful mushrooms and a custardlike polenta topping.

2¹/₂ cups water
1 cup polenta or cornmeal
10 ounces silken low-fat tofu
6 ounces Cheddar soy cheese, grated
1 large bunch spinach, washed, chopped, and drained
¹/₂ teaspoon nutmeg
1 teaspoon white pepper
¹/₂ teaspoon unrefined sea salt
1¹/₂ cups sliced wild mushrooms

Preheat the oven to 350°F.

Bring the water to a boil and slowly whisk in the polenta or cornmeal. Cook over medium heat for 5 to 10 minutes, stirring frequently.

Puree the tofu in a blender until smooth. In a medium mixing bowl, combine the tofu with the soy cheese, spinach, nutmeg, white pepper, and salt. Spread the tofu mixture into an oiled medium glass casserole. Layer the mushrooms on top of the mixture.

Top the mixture with the polenta and bake for 20 minutes or until firm and thoroughly heated. Top with Creamy White Sauce, if desired.

Fried Soba Noodles
Serves 4

In spite of its name, this recipe is a low-fat version of the traditional Japanese dish. Toasted sesame oil and ginger add extra flavor, and a little sake lessens the need for frying oil.

$^{1}/_{2}$ pound soba noodles, cooked
1 pound firm low-fat tofu, cut into $^{1}/_{2}$-inch cubes
1 medium burdock root, cut in thin slices
1 medium leek, cut in thin slices (including green tops)
2 tablespoons freshly grated ginger
$^{1}/_{2}$ cup lightly soaked hijiki
1 teaspoon light sesame oil
1 teaspoon toasted sesame oil
1 tablespoon tamari
$^{1}/_{2}$ cup sake
2 tablespoons black sesame seeds

Toss the noodles, tofu, burdock, leeks, ginger, and hijiki in a medium mixing bowl.

Heat the oils in a wok or large skillet. Add the noodle mixture and stir quickly. After the noodles are lightly coated with oil, add the tamari and sake.

Cook over medium heat for 5 to 10 minutes, or until the vegetables are tender. Add additional sake as needed while cooking to prevent sticking.

Remove from the heat and stir in the sesame seeds.

Grilled Ginger Cutlets
Serves 4 to 6

Make this tangy dish ahead of time and marinate in the refrigerator overnight. Then just add steamed greens and whole-wheat noodles for a quick and easy dinner.

1 pound firm low-fat tofu
$^1/_2$ cup tamari
$^1/_4$ cup brown rice vinegar
2 tablespoons honey
2 tablespoons finely grated fresh ginger
2 tablespoons sesame seeds
1 teaspoon toasted sesame oil
1 bunch scallions, finely sliced
1 tablespoon arrowroot powder, dissolved in a little hot water
2 tablespoons light sesame oil

Garnish
Sliced scallions and sesame seeds

Slice the tofu into cutlets, about $^1/_4$ inch thick, and layer in a casserole.

Combine the tamari, brown rice vinegar, honey, ginger, sesame seeds, and toasted sesame oil in a small bowl. Pour the marinade over the tofu slices and let the cutlets marinate overnight in the refrigerator.

Remove the cutlets from the casserole and pour the remaining marinade into a small saucepan. Add the sliced scallions and arrowroot to the marinade and cook over medium-low heat until thickened.

Heat the light sesame oil in a deep skillet and add the tofu cutlets one layer thick, turning them as they brown.

To serve, place the cutlets on a large platter, and drizzle with hot marinade. Garnish with scallions and sesame seeds.

Kale and Mushroom Casserole

Serves 4 to 6

Almost any greens can be mixed with—or substituted for—kale in this tasty recipe.

1 large bunch fresh kale or other greens, washed and chopped, with stems removed
1 tablespoon corn oil
2 cups sliced button mushrooms
1 medium red onion, chopped
1 tablespoon arrowroot, dissolved in $1/4$ cup warm water
1 teaspoon unrefined sea salt
$1/4$ cup mirin
1 cup silken low-fat tofu
$1^1/_2$ cups mozzarella-style soy cheese

Preheat the oven to 350°F.

Steam the greens just until limp. In a separate pan, heat the oil and sauté the mushrooms and onions over medium heat.

Combine the arrowroot with the salt, mirin, and tofu in a blender. Puree until smooth. Stir in the mushrooms and onions.

Combine the tofu/mushroom mixture with the greens and soy cheese. Turn the mixture into a lightly oiled large glass casserole and bake for 25 minutes.

Napa Rolls with Cashews
Makes 8 rolls

This low-fat dish, with its combination of Napa cabbage and sweet-and-sour sauce, adds an Oriental twist to an Old World favorite.

1¹/₂ cups natural vegetable burger mix
1¹/₂ cups boiling water
¹/₂ cup diced carrots
¹/₄ cup chopped cashews
¹/₄ cup currants
¹/₂ cup cooked brown rice
1 tablespoon gomashio
1 large head Napa cabbage, cored, with leaves separated

Sweet-and-Sour Sauce
¹/₂ cup honey
¹/₄ cup brown rice vinegar
2 teaspoons arrowroot, dissolved in a little warm water

Preheat the oven to 350°F.

Combine the vegetable burger mix and water and let stand 20 minutes. Add the carrots, cashews, currants, brown rice, and gomashio.

Wash the individual leaves of the Napa cabbage; steam for 1 to 2 minutes in a medium saucepan, and cool.

Roll about ¹/₂ cup of the burger mixture in 2 or 3 leaves of cabbage, and place each roll in a lightly oiled glass casserole dish, seam-side down. Bake for 20 to 30 minutes.

While the Napa rolls are baking, make the Sweet-and-Sour Sauce by combining the honey, brown rice vinegar, and arrowroot. Cook over low heat for 5 minutes, or until thick and bubbly.

Remove the rolls to a serving platter, and drizzle with Sweet-and-Sour Sauce.

Fresh Pea Pesto Noodles

Makes 4 servings

This colorful and creamy macro twist on an old classic uses green peas for a fresh-tasting pesto with a fraction of the fat.

1/2 pound soba noodles
2 cups fresh green peas
1 cup fresh chopped basil
2 tablespoons olive oil
2 tablespoons pine nuts
1/2 cup silken low-fat tofu
1 tablespoon brown rice syrup
1 teaspoon unrefined sea salt
1 teaspoon white pepper
2 cloves garlic, crushed

In a large soup pot, boil 2 quarts of water. Add the noodles and cook until just tender. Drain and rinse with cold water.

While the noodles are cooking, boil the peas in a small amount of water until tender. Drain and combine the cooked peas, basil, oil, pine nuts, tofu, brown rice syrup, salt, white pepper, and garlic in a blender, and puree until very smooth.

Add the cooked noodles to the pesto in the saucepan and stir gently until coated. Serve warm with a side dish of Honey Carrots with Caraway Seeds or Braised Radicchio and Currants.

Tofu Young

Serves 4 to 6

This vegan version of the classic Chinese favorite is an ideal meal to prepare ahead of time and store in the refrigerator—the flavors blend overnight and the pancakes turn more easily.

1 pound firm low-fat tofu
$1/2$ cup whole-wheat flour
$1/2$ cup soy milk
1 cup bean sprouts
$1/2$ cup sliced water chestnuts
$1/2$ cup finely chopped scallions
$1/2$ cup sliced shiitake mushrooms
$1/2$ cup lightly soaked hijiki
2 tablespoons tamari
2 tablespoons finely grated ginger
2 tablespoons light sesame oil
1 teaspoon toasted sesame oil
1 to 2 cups Mushroom Gravy (page 176)

Garnish
Sliced scallions

Puree the tofu with the flour and soy milk. Stir in the bean sprouts, water chestnuts, scallions, mushrooms, hijiki, tamari, and ginger. The batter should be fairly stiff—add flour if needed.

Heat the sesame oils in a deep skillet. Drop the batter by spoonfuls to form 3-inch pancakes about $1/2$ inch thick.

Cook the pancakes until golden brown, turning carefully. Serve over rice with Mushroom Gravy, and garnish with sliced scallions.

Tempura-Style Vegetables
Serves 6

This traditional Japanese dish is served at parties and on special occasions with a variety of delectable dipping sauces. Properly prepared, it shouldn't be greasy at all. Green leafy vegetables are traditionally used in tempura for their shape and texture. The leaves may be dipped in batter and deep-fried whole. Watery greens and lettuces are not recommended.

1 cup whole-wheat pastry flour
2 tablespoons arrowroot
$1/4$ teaspoon unrefined sea salt
1 cup cold water
Light sesame oil or safflower oil
$1/2$ pound button mushrooms, washed and cut in half
2 carrots, cut on the diagonal and steamed
1 cup large broccoli florets
1 medium zucchini, cut in $1/2$-inch-thick slices
1 large yellow onion, cut in $1/4$-inch-thick slices
$1/2$ pound firm low-fat tofu, cubed and dried well

Garnish
Grated daikon

Combine the flour, arrowroot, and salt, and stir in the water, mixing just until the dry ingredients are moistened. (Note: The more arrowroot you use, the thinner and crispier the tempura will be.)

Heat 2–3 inches of sesame or safflower oil in a deep frying pan or wok to about 355°F. To test the oil, drop a small bit of batter in. If the oil is the right temperature, the batter will sink and rise quickly to the top. If the batter doesn't sink, the oil is too hot; if it sinks and doesn't rise, the oil isn't hot enough.

Dip each vegetable and the cubed tofu in the batter and slide carefully into the oil, cooking until golden brown (about 1 to 3 minutes). Don't put too many vegetables in the pot at one time—doing so will lower the temperature of the oil and make the tempura soggy. About five at a time is ideal.

Remove the cooked tempura pieces with chopsticks or a slotted spoon, and set them on a rack covered with paper towels to drain. Place in a basket or on a platter covered with napkins to absorb additional oil, garnish with grated daikon, and serve with Tempura Dipping Sauce.

Where's the Meat? Loaf

Serves 6 to 8

A hearty dish with a rich, nutty flavor that makes great leftovers—just warm up slices by lightly frying in hot oil for an extra-crunchy texture.

8–10 medium carrots, chopped into 1-inch slices
$^1/_2$ cup silken tofu
$1^1/_2$ cups natural vegetable burger mix
$^1/_2$ cup oats
2 cups boiling water
$^1/_2$ cup Worcestershire sauce* or tamari
1 teaspoon black pepper
$^1/_2$ cup chopped red onions
$^1/_2$ cup sliced button mushrooms
$^1/_2$ cup pepitas
2 tablespoons sunflower oil

Preheat the oven to 350°F.

To make the carrot puree, steam the carrots in a medium saucepan in $^1/_2$ to 1 inch of water until soft. Puree with the cooking water and tofu until very smooth, thinning with additional water as needed.

Combine the burger mix, oats, and water in a large bowl. Let stand for 20 minutes. Mix the carrot puree with the Worcestershire sauce (or tamari) and black pepper in a medium bowl.

Combine the onions, mushrooms, pepitas, and carrot puree. Stir into the burger mixture. Turn into a medium loaf pan greased with sunflower oil and bake for 35 to 40 minutes. Let cool 20 minutes to set.

Slice the loaf into $^1/_2$-inch-thick portions and serve warm, with a side dish of Cauliflower Millet Mash and a bitter-greens salad.

*__Note:__ Vegetarian, preservative-free Worcestershire sauce is available at most natural products stores.

New Orleans Red Beans and Rice

Serves 4

This meat-free variation on a New Orleans favorite is a wonderful way to use leftover beans and rice. For an even more authentic taste, cook up a big pot using the made-from-scratch method.

1¹/₂ cups cooked red kidney beans
2 cups cooked brown rice
¹/₄ cup chopped fresh thyme
¹/₄ cup finely chopped fresh sage
¹/₂ teaspoon black pepper
¹/₂ teaspoon unrefined sea salt
1 tablespoon olive oil

Combine all the ingredients in a medium pot and cook over low heat until warmed through and the flavors are combined. Stir in the olive oil just before serving.

Variation: Using the made-from-scratch method, combine 1 cup soaked red kidney beans with 3 cups water in a large, heavy-bottomed pot. Bring the beans to a boil, cover, and reduce heat to low, cooking 45 minutes to 1 hour, until the beans are tender. Add 2 cups water, 1 cup short-grain brown rice, ¹/₄ cup finely chopped fresh thyme, ¹/₄ cup finely chopped fresh sage, ¹/₂ teaspoon black pepper, ¹/₂ teaspoon unrefined sea salt, and 1 tablespoon olive oil. Cook for about 30 minutes longer, or until the beans are soft and the rice is done.

Veggie Pot Pie
Serves 8

This remake of a classic American favorite is meat- and dairy-free and contains less than one-quarter the fat of the traditional recipe, with the same rich and hearty flavor.

Crust

3 cups whole-wheat pastry flour

$^1/_2$ teaspoon unrefined sea salt

$^1/_2$ cup corn or safflower oil

$^1/_2$ cup water

Pie

1 tablespoon safflower oil

$^1/_2$ cup chopped onions

$^1/_2$ cup sliced button mushrooms

1 clove garlic, minced

2 tablespoons flour

$^1/_2$ cup soy milk

1 cup Rich Vegetable Stock (see the variation of Light Vegetable Stock, page 139)

$^1/_2$ cup chopped carrots

$^1/_2$ cup peas

$^1/_2$ cup corn

$^1/_2$ cup cubed seitan

2 tablespoons each chopped fresh basil and sage

1 teaspoon black pepper

1 teaspoon unrefined sea salt

Preheat the oven to 375°F.

To make crust, combine the whole-wheat flour and salt in a large bowl. Add the corn or safflower oil and stir until the flour forms small, round balls. Mix in the cold water. Form the dough into a ball and divide in half. Roll out half the dough onto a floured surface; then place into a pie plate, pressing down the bottom and edges. Prick the crust with a fork and bake for 10 to 15 minutes. Roll out the second half of the dough for the top of the pie.

Heat the safflower oil in a medium saucepan and sauté the onions, mushrooms, and garlic until the onions are translucent. Stir in the flour and cook 1–2 minutes, stirring constantly. Slowly whisk in the soy milk and stock, and cook until thick and bubbly.

Add the carrots, peas, corn, seitan, herbs, black pepper, and salt to the mixture, and heat through.

Pour into the prebaked crust and top with the additional uncooked crust. Do not seal the edges but press lightly together. Bake for 25 minutes or until the crust is golden.

Monkfish with Sage and Roasted Red Peppers
Serves 4

This unique dish combines the delicate taste of monkfish with the distinctive flavors of browned sage and smoky roasted peppers.

2 medium red peppers
1 tablespoon safflower oil
$1/4$ cup finely chopped fresh sage
4 medium monkfish fillets, rinsed well
$1/2$ cup Light Vegetable Stock (page 139)
$1/4$ cup sake or white wine
1 teaspoon white pepper
$1/2$ teaspoon unrefined sea salt
1 tablespoon arrowroot, dissolved in $1/4$ cup warm water

Preheat the oven to 400°F.

Place the peppers on a baking sheet and cook in the oven for 30 minutes, turning several times until evenly charred on all sides. Wrap the peppers in a damp towel to cool, then cut in half and remove the stems and seeds. (Peppers may be roasted ahead of time and stored, refrigerated, in a tightly sealed container.)

Heat the oil in a medium skillet. Add the sage and cook over medium heat until slightly browned.

Add the fish to the skillet and sear on both sides. Pour in the stock and sake or white wine, and add the white pepper and salt; cover and poach the fish for about 5 minutes, or until done in the center. Remove from the pan and place on a covered serving dish.

Add the arrowroot to the mixture in the skillet and cook until thickened (about 2 minutes). Cut the roasted red peppers into long slices about $1/2$ inch wide, arrange on top of the fish, and drizzle with sauce from the pan. Serve with a wild rice mixture and Green Beans with Burdock and Mirin.

Shrimp with Cilantro Walnut Pesto
Serves 4

The pesto in this festive dish uses cilantro and walnuts instead of basil and pine nuts for a contemporary twist on the old favorite.

1 large bunch cilantro, washed well and coarsely chopped
2 tablespoons olive oil
$^1/_2$ cup chopped walnuts
2 cloves garlic, minced
1 teaspoon unrefined sea salt
$^1/_2$ teaspoon white pepper
1 pound medium shrimp, peeled, washed, and deveined
1 tablespoon safflower oil

Combine the cilantro, olive oil, walnuts, garlic, salt, and white pepper in a blender. Puree until very smooth, adding water as needed to make a thick sauce. Warm the pesto over low heat in a small saucepan.

While the pesto is warming, sauté the shrimp in the safflower oil in a medium saucepan until opaque (about 3 to 5 minutes). Serve the shrimp on noodles or rice, and drizzle pesto on top.

Ginger Plum Scallops
Serves 4 to 6

This tangy-sweet dish is a deceptively quick and easy dinner. Or increase the recipe and serve hot with toothpicks on a bed of braised field greens for a stunning but simple party appetizer.

1$^{1}/_{2}$ pounds sea scallops
1 tablespoon light sesame oil
2 tablespoons finely grated ginger
2 cloves garlic, minced
$^{1}/_{2}$ cup sake
2 tablespoons umeboshi plum paste
2 tablespoons brown rice syrup
2 tablespoons brown rice vinegar
1 teaspoon white pepper
1 tablespoon arrowroot, dissolved in $^{1}/_{4}$ cup warm water
1 cup chopped watercress

Rinse the scallops well and pat dry.

In a medium saucepan, heat the oil and add the ginger, garlic, sake, and scallops. Cook over medium-low heat for about 5 minutes.

While the scallops are cooking, combine the umeboshi plum paste, brown rice syrup, brown rice vinegar, white pepper, and arrowroot in a small bowl. Mix well.

Add the umeboshi plum sauce to the pan with the scallops and stir well to coat the scallops with sauce. Stir in the watercress and cook for 5 more minutes, or until the watercress is limp and the scallops are cooked through. Serve over brown rice or udon noodles.

Cinnamon Sole
Serves 4

The unexpected combination of sweet and spicy, hot and cold, makes this a perfect party offering or a main dish for special dinners. Serve over basmati rice with a simple side dish of steamed green vegetables.

4 fillets of sole
1 tablespoon cinnamon
1 to 2 teaspoons cayenne pepper
1 tablespoon almond or corn oil
$1/2$ cup Light Vegetable Stock (page 139)
$1/2$ cup soy milk
1 tablespoon arrowroot, dissolved in $1/4$ cup warm water
1 ripe peach, thinly sliced
1 small apple, thinly sliced and poached

Rinse the fish fillets well and pat dry. Combine the cinnamon and cayenne pepper in a small bowl, then spread onto a plate. Coat each fillet with the cinnamon mixture.

In a medium skillet, heat the oil over medium-high heat. Add the fish and sear on both sides. Pour in the stock; cover the skillet and poach until the fish is flaky and tender. Remove the fish carefully to serving dish.

Combine the soy milk and arrowroot, add to the stock in the skillet, and cook until thickened (about 2 minutes). Arrange the sliced fruit on top of the fish, and pour the sauce over the fillets and fruit.

Honey Ginger Shrimp and Udon
Serves 4

This deceptively simple but decidedly gourmet dish makes a low-fat weekday meal or dinner party dish.

6 cups water
$^1/_2$ pound udon noodles
1 teaspoon light sesame oil
1 teaspoon toasted sesame oil
1 medium leek, thinly sliced (including green top)
$^1/_2$ cup sliced button mushrooms
$^1/_4$ cup grated ginger
1 pound medium shrimp, peeled and deveined
$^1/_4$ cup honey
2 tablespoons gomashio
$^1/_4$ cup tamari

Bring the water to a boil in a large pot. Add the udon noodles and cook 8 to 10 minutes, or just until tender. Drain and set aside.

Heat the oils in a medium saucepan and sauté the leeks, mushrooms, and ginger until the leeks are translucent. Add the shrimp and sauté over medium heat until the shrimp are just done (about 5 minutes).

Stir in the honey, gomashio, and tamari. Toss with the noodles, and serve either hot or cold.

14

VEGETABLES
AND SIDE DISHES

Hearty Corn and Asparagus Stir-Fry
Serves 6

The hearty taste of tempeh combines with delicate asparagus and corn for a most unusual dish.

1 tablespoon almond or corn oil
1 small yellow onion, chopped
$^1/_2$ teaspoon unrefined sea salt
1 (8-ounce) package tempeh, crumbled
2 tablespoons tamari
2 cups fresh corn kernels
2 cups asparagus, cut into 1-inch sections
$^1/_4$ teaspoon black pepper
$^1/_4$ cup chopped almonds
$^1/_4$ cup water
1 tablespoon brown rice syrup

Heat the oil in a medium saucepan. Add the onions and salt and sauté until the onions are translucent. Stir in the tempeh and tamari, and cook until the tempeh is lightly browned and crunchy.

Add the corn, asparagus, black pepper, almonds, water, and brown rice syrup, stirring well to combine all the ingredients. Cook over medium heat for 5 minutes longer, or until the corn is just done.

Red Cabbage and Peas with Cumin Seed

Serves 6

A zesty way to serve plain old cabbage. This dish, with its Indian twist, goes especially well with Poppyseed Onion Chapati and makes a wonderful leftover lunch—try it chilled with a splash of brown rice vinegar.

1 tablespoon olive oil
1 medium head red cabbage, shredded
2 cups fresh green peas
$1/2$ teaspoon unrefined sea salt
$1/4$ cup water
$1/2$ teaspoon cumin seeds
$1/2$ teaspoon caraway seeds

Heat the oil in a large saucepan. Add the cabbage and peas, sprinkle with salt, and stir until the vegetables are evenly coated with oil.

Add the water, cover, and cook for about 5 minutes, or until the cabbage is tender.

Lightly crush the cumin and caraway seeds in a suribachi or spice mill. Add to the cabbage mixture and cook for 3 to 5 minutes longer.

Brussels Sprouts with Shiitake Mushrooms

Serves 4

Even the fussiest feeders will enjoy this flavorful preparation of Brussels sprouts.

$1^{1}/2$ pounds Brussels sprouts, halved, with stems removed
2 teaspoons light sesame oil
$1/2$ cup sliced shiitake mushrooms
$1/4$ teaspoon unrefined sea salt
$1/2$ cup grated carrots
$1/4$ cup sake
2 tablespoons brown rice syrup
$1/4$ cup sesame seeds

Drop the sprouts into 1 inch of boiling water and cook for about 5 minutes; drain well.

While the sprouts are cooking, heat the oil in a large skillet and sauté the mushrooms with salt until the mushrooms wilt. Add the parboiled sprouts and cook over medium heat 5 minutes longer.

Stir in the carrots, sake, brown rice syrup, and sesame seeds. Cook 5 minutes longer, until the glaze thickens and the sprouts are tender.

Braised Radicchio and Currants
Serves 4 to 6

Currants and brown rice syrup add a new twist to this still-trendy member of the chicory family.

2 medium heads radicchio
2 teaspoons almond or olive oil
$1/2$ cup currants
2 tablespoons brown rice syrup

Cut each radicchio head into 8 to 12 wedges, removing the core.

Heat the oil in a medium skillet and add the radicchio wedges and currants.

Cook over medium heat just until the radicchio wilts. Add the brown rice syrup and stir to coat well.

Butternut Squash with Sprouted Sunflower Seeds
Serves 4

This warming winter side dish is wonderful as a lunchtime leftover, spread on flat bread or rolled in leaves of lightly steamed greens.

1 medium butternut squash, cut into cubes
1 medium yellow onion, diced
3 tablespoons mellow white miso
3 tablespoons sunflower butter
$1/2$ cup sprouted sunflower seeds
$1/4$ cup finely chopped parsley

Steam the squash in a large saucepan for about 20 minutes, or until soft. Add the onions during last 5 minutes.

Combine the squash mixture with the miso and sunflower butter. Pour into a blender and puree until very smooth.

Return the squash mixture to the pan and add the sprouts and parsley. Heat gently, and serve as a side dish with any meal.

Note: To sprout sunflower seeds, soak 1 cup seeds in 2 cups cool water overnight. Drain the soaking water the next morning and allow seeds to sprout for about 24 hours, or just until small "nubs" appear at the end of the seeds.

Steamed Fennel Wedges
Serves 4

The anise undertones and dark purple color of fresh opal basil are the perfect complements for this often forgotten vegetable.

4 small to medium fennel bulbs
1 tablespoon olive oil
$1/2$ teaspoon unrefined sea salt
$1/4$ cup chopped opal or regular basil

Wash the fennel bulbs, pat dry, and cut into quarters.

Heat the oil in a large saucepan. Add the quartered fennel and salt, and toss to lightly coat. Cook over medium heat until the fennel begins to sweat, then add $1/2$ inch of water and cover, cooking until tender.

Add the basil just before serving, and heat until it wilts.

Green Beans with Burdock and Mirin
Serves 4

Fresh green beans make a light, colorful side dish for any meal, and the flavors of burdock and mirin add extra interest.

2 teaspoons safflower oil
1 pound green beans, washed, with stems removed
$1/2$ teaspoon unrefined sea salt
1 medium burdock root, washed well and thinly sliced on the diagonal
2 tablespoons finely grated ginger
$1/2$ cup mirin
2 tablespoons sesame seeds

Heat the oil in a medium saucepan over medium flame. Add the green beans and salt, stirring to coat well. Lower the heat and cook about 5 minutes, stirring often.

Add the burdock, ginger, and mirin, stirring well to combine. Cover and cook over medium heat (adding water as needed to prevent sticking) until the burdock is tender (5–7 minutes).

Stir in the sesame seeds, and serve hot or at room temperature as a salad.

Appled Beets
Serves 4

Everyone loves beets cooked this way. Try cutting leftovers into slivers and adding them to tossed green salads.

1 pound beets
¹/₂ cup apple juice
2 tablespoons brown rice vinegar
2 tablespoons poppyseeds
1 tablespoon finely chopped parsley

Scrub the beets well; peel and cut into thin (¹/₈-inch) slices.

Pour the apple juice into a medium pan. Add the beets, cover, and cook until tender.

Stir in the brown rice vinegar and poppyseeds, and heat through. Add the parsley just before serving.

Honey Carrots with Caraway Seeds
Serves 4

The pungent flavors of caraway and balsamic vinegar complement the sweet carrots and honey in this colorful side dish.

1 pound carrots
1 teaspoon sunflower oil
1 teaspoon unrefined sea salt
¹/₄ cup honey
2 tablespoons brown rice or balsamic vinegar
2 tablespoons caraway seeds

Scrub the carrots well and cut into ¹/₄-inch-thick diagonal slices.

Heat the oil in a medium pan. Add the carrots and salt, and toss to lightly coat with oil. Cook over medium-low heat until the carrots begin to sweat. Cover and cook over low until the carrots are tender, adding a small amount of water if needed to prevent sticking.

Add the honey, vinegar, and caraway seeds just before serving.

Cauliflower Millet Mash
Serves 6

An intriguing alternative to mashed potatoes, this creamy combination of flavors provides a more nutritious, tastier side dish. Garnish with sprigs of fresh parsley for color.

$^1/_2$ cup millet
$1^1/_2$ cups water
1 medium head cauliflower, chopped
1 teaspoon unrefined sea salt
$^1/_4$ cup tahini

In a medium saucepan, dry toast the millet over medium-high heat until it turns a deep golden color. Add the water. Lower the heat, cover, and cook until all the water is absorbed (about 20 to 30 minutes).

While the millet is cooking, steam the cauliflower until very soft (about 10 minutes).

Combine the cooked millet and cauliflower in a blender and puree until smooth. Add the salt and tahini, and puree again until creamy.

Parsnip Puree
Serves 4 to 6

Creamy and rich, this satisfying side dish combines the unexpected, delicately sweet flavor of parsnips with carrots and cauliflower. For a nutty flavor, add a little tahini.

$^1/_2$ teaspoon unrefined sea salt
2 cups sliced parsnips
$1^1/_2$ cups sliced carrots
1 cup cauliflower florets
$^1/_2$ pound silken low-fat tofu
$^1/_2$ teaspoon white pepper
$^1/_2$ teaspoon nutmeg
$^1/_4$ cup tahini (optional)

In a large pot, heat 1 inch of water to boiling; add the salt, parsnips, carrots, and cauliflower, and steam until very tender.

Drain the vegetables and puree with the tofu, white pepper, nutmeg, and tahini (if desired) in a blender. Serve hot.

Winter Vegetable Bake
Serves 6 to 8

A low-fat, incredibly satisfying side dish. Make enough for lunch leftovers—they reheat easily and are wonderful at room temperature as well.

1 medium butternut squash, peeled and cut into 1-inch cubes
2 medium red onions, cut into wedges
6 to 8 carrots, cut on the diagonal in $1/2$-inch-thick slices
3 large turnips, cut into 1-inch cubes
2 medium rutabagas, cut into 1-inch cubes
5 parsnips, cut on the diagonal in $1/2$-inch-thick slices
8 garlic cloves, peeled
1 bunch fresh rosemary, chopped, with stems removed
1 teaspoon white pepper
1 teaspoon unrefined sea salt
1–2 tablespoons olive oil

Preheat the oven to 400°F.

Toss the vegetables in a large mixing bowl with the rosemary, white pepper, and salt to coat.

Spread out evenly, one layer thick, on one or two large cookie sheets. Drizzle with olive oil.

Bake until the vegetables are tender but still firm (about 25 minutes), stirring frequently. Serve immediately.

Wild Rice Pesto

Serves 4

A low-fat, savory pesto transforms chewy, nutty wild rice into a unique side serving or perfect party dish.

4 cups water
1 cup wild rice
1 cup short-grain brown rice
1 tablespoon olive oil
1 medium yellow onion, chopped
1/2 teaspoon unrefined sea salt
1/2 teaspoon white pepper
2 teaspoons whole-wheat flour
1/2 cup water
1/2 pound silken low-fat tofu, mashed
2 cups chopped fresh basil
1/2 cup pine nuts

Bring the 4 cups water to a boil in a large pot. Add the wild and brown rices. Cover, then lower the heat and simmer until the rice is soft (45 minutes to 1 hour).

Heat the oil in a medium saucepan and sauté the onions with the salt and white pepper until the onions are translucent.

Add the flour and stir until the onions are well coated. Cook for 2 minutes; stir in the 1/2 cup water and tofu, and blend over medium heat until smooth and creamy. Add the basil and pine nuts; puree mixture until smooth.

Stir in the rice, heat through, and serve.

Roots and Greens Casserole
Serves 6 to 8

The unique combination of flavors and textures in this savory casserole is even better the next day. Try making it ahead of time for a quicker fix and to let the flavors blend.

2 tablespoons sunflower oil
1 bunch Swiss chard, washed, with stems removed
2 large sweet potatoes, cut into $1/4$-inch slices
4 medium parsnips, cut into $1/4$-inch slices
1 medium yellow onion, sliced
1 teaspoon cardamom
1 teaspoon nutmeg
1 teaspoon unrefined sea salt
1 cup Creamy White Sauce (page 175)

Preheat the oven to 375°F.

Lightly grease the bottom of a large glass casserole with the oil. Layer with half of the Swiss chard leaves.

Layer the sweet potatoes on top of the Swiss chard. Add another layer of chard, then layer the parsnips and onions on top. Sprinkle with cardamom, nutmeg, and salt.

Cover the casserole loosely with foil and bake for 20 minutes. Pour the Creamy White Sauce over the vegetables and continue baking for 10 minutes, or until the sweet potatoes are tender. Sprinkle with fresh grated nutmeg before serving.

Red Peppers in Mirin
Serves 4 to 6

The delicately sweet taste of mirin is the perfect complement to red peppers and pine nuts.

4 medium red peppers, cut into $1/4$-inch-wide strips
$1/4$ cup mirin
$1/4$ cup sake
$1/2$ teaspoon unrefined sea salt
$1/2$ teaspoon black pepper
$1/4$ cup pine nuts
$1/2$ cup fresh chopped basil

In a medium saucepan, combine the peppers, mirin, sake, salt, and black pepper. Cover and simmer gently until the peppers are tender (about 5 minutes).

Stir in the pine nuts and basil, and cook for 2 minutes longer, or until the basil is wilted.

Acorn Squash with Barley
Serves 4

The meatlike texture of frozen tofu gives this hearty winter dish a richer, more substantial taste. Serve with a light miso soup and leafy greens for a complete meal.

2 medium acorn squash
2 tablespoons safflower oil
$1/2$ cup firm tofu, frozen and then defrosted, drained well, and crumbled
$1/2$ cup thinly sliced scallions (including green tops)
$1/2$ cup lightly soaked hijiki
1 cup cooked barley

Preheat the oven to 375°F.
Scrub the squash, cut in half, and scoop out the seeds.
In a medium skillet, heat the oil and add the crumbled tofu and scallions. Cook over medium heat until the tofu is browned and the scallions are translucent (about 5 minutes).
Add the hijiki to the tofu mixture. Stir the tofu mixture into the cooked barley, and spoon into the squash halves. Bake for 30 to 40 minutes, or until the squash is tender.

Beans and Greens
Serves 4

Try this Southern favorite as a quick party dish or light dinner, served with Creamy Southern Spoonbread.

1 tablespoon olive oil
1 medium red onion, chopped
$^1/_2$ teaspoon unrefined sea salt
$^1/_2$ teaspoon black pepper
1 large bunch collard greens, coarsely chopped
$^1/_4$ cup water
2 cups cooked black-eyed peas
$1^1/_2$ tablespoons brown rice vinegar

Heat the oil in a medium saucepan and sauté the onions, salt, and black pepper until the onions are translucent.

Stir in the collard greens and water, cover tightly, and steam over medium heat until the greens are bright green and limp (about 3–5 minutes). Add the peas and cook for 5 more minutes to allow the flavors to blend.

Spoon into individual bowls or plates, and float 1 teaspoonful of vinegar on each portion just before serving.

Creamy Southern Spoonbread
Makes 8 servings

The crunchy texture of whole corn kernels adds a novel surprise to this soft and creamy low-fat take on a traditional Southern favorite.

2 cups soy milk
2 tablespoons brown rice vinegar
$1/2$ pound silken low-fat tofu
2 teaspoons brown rice syrup
3 cups cornmeal
1 cup unbleached flour
1 teaspoon unrefined sea salt
2 cups corn kernels
1 cup finely chopped onion

Preheat the oven to 375°F.

In a medium bowl, combine the soy milk with the brown rice vinegar and let sit for 5 minutes. Puree with the tofu and brown rice syrup until very smooth.

Combine the cornmeal, flour, and salt in a large mixing bowl.

Combine the corn kernels and onion with the soy milk mixture in a medium bowl, and beat well. Pour the corn and soy milk mixture into the flour mixture, and stir gently until the ingredients are moistened. Pour into a cast-iron skillet or an 8-inch-square casserole coated with safflower oil.

Bake for 30 to 40 minutes. Let cool slightly and spoon out to serve (the bread should be slightly soft and custardlike in the center).

15

DRESSINGS AND SAUCES

Creamy White Sauce
Makes 2 cups

A versatile vegan version of the traditional favorite. Add fresh or dried herbs of your choice to vary the flavor for different dishes.

3 tablespoons corn or sunflower oil
3 tablespoons whole-wheat flour
1 cup soy milk
1 teaspoon white pepper
1 teaspoon unrefined sea salt
$1/2$ cup Light Vegetable Stock (page 139)
$1/2$ cup sake or white wine
Unrefined sea salt, white or black pepper, herbs (optional)

Heat the oil in a medium skillet. Stir in the flour and cook over medium to low heat for 1 to 2 minutes, being careful not to brown the flour.

Slowly whisk in the soy milk, white pepper, salt, and stock. Cook for 2 to 3 minutes longer, or until thick and bubbly.

Remove from the heat and whisk in the sake or wine. Add other herbs or spices to taste, if desired.

Mushroom Gravy

Makes 3 cups

This rich, versatile sauce has surprisingly little fat—the secret is in using mature mushrooms and a highly seasoned stock. For more exotic variations, try shiitake mushrooms, or substitute chanterelles or morels for a portion of the button mushrooms.

2 tablespoons olive oil
3 cups finely chopped mushrooms
1 medium onion, chopped
1 teaspoon unrefined sea salt
1 teaspoon black pepper
3 tablespoons flour
3/4 cup soy milk
3/4 cup Rich Vegetable Stock (see variation of Light Vegetable Stock, page 139)
2 tablespoons finely chopped fresh sage (optional)

Heat the oil in a large saucepan. Add the mushrooms, onion, salt, and black pepper, and sauté until the mushrooms are soft.

Add the flour and stir until the mushrooms are coated. Cook over low heat for 2 to 3 minutes, stirring constantly.

Slowly stir in the soy milk and stock. Cook for 2 to 5 minutes longer, or until thick and bubbly.

Transfer the mixture to a blender, and puree on high speed, leaving some mushroom chunks for texture. Add chopped sage if desired.

Peanut Ginger Dressing
Makes 3 cups

Ginger teams up with peanut butter to make a nutty, versatile dressing. Serve it cold on salads, warmed over noodles, or as a dipping sauce for fried tempeh.

1 cup natural peanut butter
1 cup warm water
$1/4$ pound silken low-fat tofu
$1/2$ cup grated ginger
2 tablespoons tamari
2 tablespoons brown rice syrup
2 tablespoons gomashio

Puree all the ingredients in a blender until smooth. Chill before serving to allow the flavors to blend.

Miso Umeboshi Sauce
Makes 1 cup

This tangy, versatile combination doubles as a dressing or sauce for seafood or noodle dishes.

2 tablespoons toasted sesame oil
2 tablespoons tamari
$1/4$ cup brown rice syrup
2 tablespoons brown rice vinegar
1 tablespoon arrowroot, dissolved in $1/4$ cup warm water
1 tablespoon umeboshi plum paste
2 tablespoons white miso
$1/4$ cup warm water
1 tablespoon gomashio

Combine the oil, tamari, brown rice syrup, and brown rice vinegar in a small saucepan. Bring to a slow boil, then add the arrowroot mixture.

Let the mixture simmer for 5 minutes, until thick and bubbly, then remove from the heat and let it sit to thicken.

Combine the umeboshi and miso with warm water to thin. Stir into the tamari mixture and mix until smooth. Add the gomashio and cool.

Red Pepper Puree
Makes 2 cups

Use this smoky, slightly sweet sauce as a dressing or in place of tomato sauce in many recipes. Try substituting yellow bell peppers for a milder flavor.

4 medium red peppers
1 tablespoon olive oil
¹/₂ teaspoon white pepper
¹/₂ teaspoon unrefined sea salt
1–2 teaspoons brown rice syrup
Finely chopped fresh basil, rosemary, sage, or other herbs (optional)

Preheat the oven to 400°F.

Place the peppers on a baking sheet and bake for 30 to 45 minutes, turning several times until evenly charred on all sides. Wrap the peppers in a damp towel to cool, then cut in half and remove the stems and seeds.

Combine the roasted peppers with the olive oil, white pepper, salt, and rice syrup in a blender. Puree until very smooth.

Add a handful of chopped herbs if desired, and blend well with the sauce.

Creamy Ginger Dressing
Makes 2 cups

The pungent flavors of garlic and ginger make this savory salad dressing a perfect addition to cold greens and grains. Or use it warmed and drizzled over vegetables.

4 cloves garlic, crushed
¹/₄ cup grated ginger
¹/₄ cup tamari
¹/₄ cup tahini
¹/₄ cup water
2 tablespoons mellow white miso
2 tablespoons brown rice syrup
1 bunch scallions, thinly sliced (including green tops)
1 tablespoon gomashio

Puree the garlic, ginger, tamari, tahini, water, miso, and brown rice syrup in a blender until very smooth. Stir in the scallions and gomashio. Before serving, chill until the flavors are well blended.

Raspberry Poppyseed Vinaigrette
Makes 1 cup

The slightly sweet but tangy flavor of this healthy alternative to cream-based dressings is perfect on bitter lettuces or mixed field greens.

$1/4$ cup raspberry vinegar
$1/2$ cup walnut or almond oil
$1/4$ cup natural raspberry jam or preserves
$1/2$ teaspoon unrefined sea salt
1 tablespoon poppyseeds

Combine all the ingredients in a small mixing bowl and blend until the preserves are smooth. Chill well to let the flavors blend, and serve at room temperature.

Sunflower Peach Dressing
Makes 1 cup

Sweet and light with a fresh, delicate flavor, this dressing is a perfect balance for bitter-greens salads.

1 large, very ripe peach
2 tablespoons sunflower butter
1 tablespoon brown rice syrup
1 teaspoon mellow white miso
2 tablespoons brown rice vinegar
$1/2$ cup peach or apple juice
$1/4$ cup sprouted sunflower seeds
Unrefined sea salt to taste

Chop the peach into small chunks. Combine with the sunflower butter, brown rice syrup, miso, vinegar, and juice in a blender, and puree until smooth.

Stir in the sunflower seeds and salt, and add extra juice as needed to thin. Chill thoroughly before serving.

Raisin Peach Chutney
Makes 3 cups

Serve chilled or at room temperature with chapatis or vegetable fritters as a savory dipping sauce, or use as a marinade for special fish dishes.

1 cup raisins
$^1/_4$ cup unsweetened, shredded coconut
1 large, very ripe peach, mashed
$^1/_2$ cup brown rice syrup
$^1/_2$ cup brown rice vinegar

Combine all the ingredients in a heavy saucepan.

Bring to a full boil, then simmer 10–15 minutes until thick, stirring frequently. Chill or serve at room temperature.

Apple Basil Vinaigrette
Makes 2 cups

This low-fat, fresh dressing is the consummate complement to a sprouted salad of lentils, azuki beans, and sunflower seeds.

1 large apple
2 tablespoons brown rice syrup
2 tablespoons mellow white miso
2 tablespoons brown rice vinegar
2 tablespoons olive oil
$^1/_4$ cup apple juice
$^1/_2$ cup chopped basil
$^1/_4$ cup finely chopped walnuts
Unrefined sea salt to taste

Core the apple and chop into small chunks. Combine with the brown rice syrup, miso, brown rice vinegar, oil, and apple juice in a blender, and puree until smooth.

Stir in the basil, walnuts, and salt, and add extra apple juice as needed to thin. Chill thoroughly before serving.

Tempura Dipping Sauce
Makes 1¹/₂ cups

This traditional dipping sauce is designed to balance the taste of tempura and make the oil more digestible.

¹/₂ cup tamari
¹/₂ cup Kombu Dashi Stock (page 139)
¹/₄ cup grated ginger
2 tablespoons grated daikon
2 tablespoons mirin
2 tablespoons thinly sliced scallions

Combine all the ingredients, and serve in individual dipping bowls with Tempura-Style Vegetables.

Ginger Garlic Sauce
Makes 1 cup

Try using olive oil instead of sesame oil and substituting fresh basil or oregano for the ginger to add an Italian twist to this versatile sauce.

2 tablespoons light sesame oil
3 cloves fresh garlic, minced
3 tablespoons finely grated ginger
2 tablespoons whole-wheat flour
¹/₂ cup Kombu Dashi Stock (page 139)
¹/₂ cup soy milk
1 teaspoon white pepper
¹/₂ teaspoon unrefined sea salt

In a medium saucepan, heat the oil and sauté the garlic and ginger until soft but not browned.

Add the flour and stir to coat the garlic and ginger. Cook for 2 to 3 minutes, stirring frequently; then slowly stir in the stock and soy milk, cooking over low heat for 5 minutes longer, or until the sauce is thick and the flavors are well blended.

Add the white pepper and salt, and serve over udon noodles or steamed vegetables.

Almond Cream
Makes 1¹/₂ cups

A sweet treat that makes a creamy, rich addition to any fruit dessert. Use a dollop on fruit compotes or baked apples.

1 (10-ounce) package silken tofu
¹/₂ cup brown rice syrup
¹/₂ cup almond butter
1 tablespoon vanilla extract

Combine all the ingredients in a blender, and puree until very smooth. Pour into a glass container and chill.

Tahini Apple Butter
Makes 1¹/₂ cups

Drizzle this creamy concoction over summer fruit salads, or spread lightly on warm muffins or pancakes for a luscious, healthy breakfast treat.

1 cup chopped apple
¹/₄ cup tahini
¹/₄ cup brown rice syrup
2 teaspoons vanilla

Combine all the ingredients in a blender, and puree until creamy and smooth. Store in a tightly sealed glass container in the refrigerator.

Apple Raisin Syrup

Makes 2 cups

A versatile, healthy sweetener that's a wonderful alternative to maple syrup on morning pancakes.

1¹/₂ cups natural applesauce, chunky style
1 tablespoon arrowroot, dissolved in ¹/₄ cup water
¹/₄ cup brown rice syrup
¹/₂ cup raisins
1 teaspoon cinnamon

Combine all the ingredients in a small saucepan. Bring to a slow boil, then let the mixture simmer for 5 minutes. Remove from the heat and let sit to thicken.

Blueberry Sauce

Makes 2 cups

Try drizzling this colorful concoction on breakfast cereals or morning muffins instead of using butter or jam.

1¹/₂ cups fresh blueberries
¹/₄ cup rice milk
¹/₂ cup brown rice syrup
1 tablespoon arrowroot, dissolved in ¹/₄ cup water
¹/₂ teaspoon vanilla

Puree the blueberries and rice milk in a blender until smooth.

Combine the blueberry mixture, brown rice syrup, and arrowroot mixture in a small saucepan. Bring to a slow boil, then let the mixture simmer for 5 minutes. Remove from the heat, stir in the vanilla, and let sit to thicken. Store in a tightly sealed glass container.

16

QUICK FIXES
Breakfast on the Go

Sunny Roll-Ups
Serves 4 to 6

1 cup oats
1 cup whole-wheat flour
$^1/_2$ teaspoon unrefined sea salt
$^1/_2$ cup sunflower seeds
1$^1/_2$ cups soy milk
$^1/_2$ cup apple juice
1–2 tablespoons sunflower oil

Filling
$^1/_4$ cup sunflower butter
$^1/_4$ cup brown rice syrup

Combine the dry ingredients in a medium bowl and add the soy milk and apple juice. The mixture should be fairly thin—if necessary, add a little water or apple juice. Lightly coat a large skillet with the sunflower oil; heat over medium flame and pour the mixture by large spoonfuls onto the skillet to make thin pancakes. Brown lightly on both sides, remove to a platter, and let cool.

Combine the sunflower butter and brown rice syrup; spread each pancake with filling and roll up. Serve whole or cut into pinwheels and arrange on a serving platter.

Mixed-Grain Breakfast Blend
Serves 4

3 cups leftover cooked rice, oats, barley, millet, or other grain
1 cup soy or rice milk
$1/2$ cup raisins, chopped dried apricots, or chopped dried apples
$1/4$ cup sesame seeds or sunflower seeds
3 tablespoons brown rice syrup or barley malt syrup
1 teaspoon vanilla extract

Combine all ingredients in medium saucepan and heat over low flame until creamy and warmed through (about 5 minutes).

Berry Crunch with Soy Yogurt
Serves 4 to 6

2 cups blueberries or raspberries
2 medium, very ripe pears, thinly sliced
2 medium peaches
$1/4$ cup brown rice syrup
$1/4$ cup sunflower oil
1 cup uncooked oats
1 cup soy yogurt
1 teaspoon vanilla
2 teaspoons honey

Preheat the oven to 350°F.

Combine the berries, pears, and peaches, and layer in a medium glass casserole dish. Combine the brown rice syrup, oil, and oats, and sprinkle on the top of the fruit. Bake for 15 to 20 minutes, or until bubbly. Combine the yogurt, vanilla, and honey, and drizzle the yogurt mixture over the compote.

Tahini Spread
Makes 2 cups

1 cup leftover cooked winter squash
$1/4$ cup tahini
$1/4$ cup brown rice syrup
$1/4$ cup sesame seeds

Combine the squash, tahini, and brown rice syrup in a blender, and puree until smooth. Stir in sesame seeds. Spread on pancake roll-ups, chapati, tortillas, or unleavened bread.

Whole-Grain Pancakes
Serves 4 to 6

$^1/_2$ cup leftover cooked rice, millet, or barley
$^1/_2$ cup raw oats
1 cup whole-grain flour
$^1/_2$ teaspoon unrefined sea salt
$^1/_4$ cup pecans
2 tablespoons barley malt syrup
$1^1/_2$ cups soy milk
$^1/_2$ teaspoon vanilla or cinnamon (optional)
1–2 tablespoons sunflower oil

Syrup
$^1/_4$ cup apple juice
$^1/_2$ cup brown rice syrup
$^1/_4$ cup tahini

Combine the grains and dry ingredients in a medium bowl. Mix the barley malt syrup, soy milk, and vanilla or cinnamon (optional) until well blended, then stir into the dry mixture. Let sit for about 15 minutes.

Lightly coat a large skillet with the sunflower oil; heat over medium flame and drop the mixture by large spoonfuls onto the skillet, browning on both sides.

To make the syrup, combine the juice and rice syrup in a small pot, and heat over a medium flame until the mixture begins to thicken. Stir in the tahini and remove from the heat. Drizzle the sauce over the pancakes, and garnish with fresh fruit slices.

Baked Apples with Raisins and Cinnamon
Serves 4

4 apples, thinly sliced
2 tablespoons honey
$^1/_2$ teaspoon cinnamon
$^1/_4$ cup raisins

Preheat the oven to 350°F.

Add $^1/_4$ inch water to a small glass casserole dish. Layer the apple slices in the casserole. Combine the honey, cinnamon, and raisins, and drizzle over the apples. Bake for 15 minutes.

Country Breakfast Scramble
Makes 4 to 6 servings

A cholesterol- and dairy-free alternative to the bacon-and-eggs breakfast routine. Try stuffing leftovers in pita pockets with crunchy sprouts for a quick and easy, nutritious lunch.

1 pound firm low-fat tofu, frozen and thawed
1 teaspoon turmeric
2 teaspoons corn oil
$1/2$ cup chopped red onions
$1/2$ cup sliced button mushrooms
$1/4$ cup chopped fresh tarragon
$1/2$ teaspoon unrefined sea salt
$1/2$ teaspoon black pepper

Drain the tofu well and crumble into a medium mixing bowl. Add the turmeric and stir until well blended.

Heat the oil in a medium skillet and sauté the onions and mushrooms until the onions are translucent. Stir in the tarragon, salt, and black pepper.

Add the tofu and cook for 3 to 5 minutes.

Note: $1/2$ cup soy cheese may be added at the end of cooking, if desired.

Millet Porridge
Serves 4 to 6

1 cup rice milk
1 cup leftover cooked winter squash
2 cups cooked millet
$1/4$ cup apple juice
$1/4$ cup barley malt syrup
$1/4$ teaspoon unrefined sea salt
$1/2$ cup almonds

Combine the rice milk and squash in a blender, and puree until smooth. Stir into the millet, thinning with apple juice as needed. Add barley malt syrup, salt, and almonds, and cook over medium heat in a medium saucepan until thick and bubbly.

Breakfast Smoothie
Serves 4

2 cups rice or soy milk
1 cup apple juice
1 cup blueberries, raspberries, or strawberries
2 ripe bananas
1 tablespoon brown rice syrup

Combine all the ingredients in a blender, and puree until smooth. Serve garnished with berries or slices of banana.

Sweet Potatoes with Pecans
Serves 4

2 cups cooked sweet potatoes, cubed
$1/4$ cup chopped dried apricots
$1/4$ cup barley malt syrup
$1/4$ cup pecans
$1/4$ cup apple juice

Combine all the ingredients in a medium saucepan, and stir until well coated. Cook over medium heat until the vegetables are very soft and the mixture becomes bubbly. Serve hot.

Berry Nut Compote
Serves 4 to 6

2 teaspoons sunflower oil
1 cup leftover cooked millet
1 cup leftover cooked rice, barley, or other grain
$1/2$ cup uncooked oats
$1/2$ cup almonds, pecans, or sunflower seeds
1 cup blueberries
1 cup peaches

Preheat the oven to 350°F.
   Coat a medium casserole with the oil. Combine the grains and nuts, and press firmly into a medium casserole, lining the bottom and sides. Combine the fruit and spread evenly onto the grain crust. Bake for 15 minutes.

17

JUST DESSERTS

Berry Peach Tart with Oatmeal Crunch
Serves 8 to 10

1$^1/_2$ cups whole-wheat pastry flour
$^3/_4$ cup whole oats
$^1/_2$ teaspoon unrefined sea salt
$^1/_2$ cup safflower oil
$^1/_2$ cup apple juice
3 cups fresh, thinly sliced peaches
1 cup blueberries
2 tablespoons whole-wheat flour
$^1/_2$ cup brown rice syrup
$^1/_4$ cup sunflower oil

Preheat the oven to 375°F.

Combine the pastry flour, $^1/_2$ cup oats, salt, and oil. Stir in the apple juice with a fork, form into a ball, and roll out on a lightly floured surface. Press into a 9-inch pie pan. Gently mix the fruit with the whole-wheat flour and $^1/_4$ cup brown rice syrup. Pour into the crust. Combine the remaining oats and brown rice syrup with the oil; mix well and crumble over the fruit filling. Bake for 35 minutes, or until the fruit is soft and juicy and the oat topping is lightly browned.

Pumpkin Pudding
Serves 4

2 cups cooked pumpkin (or other winter squash)
1 block silken tofu
$1/4$ cup barley malt syrup
$1/4$ teaspoon unrefined sea salt
Rice milk as needed

Puree all the ingredients until creamy and smooth, adding rice milk as needed to thin. Pour into individual dishes, chill, and serve cool.

Tahini Vanilla Cookies
Makes 4 dozen cookies

$1/2$ cup tahini
$3/4$ cup brown rice syrup
1 teaspoon vanilla
$1^{1}/2$ cups whole-wheat flour
$1/2$ cup whole oats
$1/4$ teaspoon unrefined sea salt
$1/4$ cup sesame seeds
$1/4$ cup finely chopped walnuts
$1/2$ cup soy milk

Preheat the oven to 350°F.

Beat the tahini, brown rice syrup, and vanilla until smooth and creamy. Mix the flour, oats, salt, sesame seeds, and walnuts in a large bowl. Stir in the tahini mixture and soy milk, and blend well. Drop by rounded spoonfuls onto a lightly oiled cookie sheet, pressing down to form $1/4$-inch-thick cookies. Bake for 10 to 15 minutes.

Apples with Almond Cream

Serves 4

4 medium apples, thinly sliced
$1/4$ cup apple juice
$1/4$ cup almonds
2 tablespoons barley malt syrup
1 block silken tofu
$1/4$ cup almond butter
$1/4$ cup brown rice syrup

Place the apples and juice in a medium saucepan, cover tightly, and boil until tender. Drain off excess liquid and reserve; stir in the almonds and barley malt syrup. Puree the tofu with cooking liquid, almond butter, and brown rice syrup until creamy. Spoon the apples into individual serving dishes, and top with a dollop of the almond cream.

Millet Custard

Serves 4 to 6

3 cups cooked millet
1 cup soy milk
$1/2$ cup chopped walnuts
$1/2$ teaspoon cinnamon
$1/4$ cup brown rice syrup

Combine all the ingredients and cook until creamy. Serve warm or pour into individual serving dishes and chill, then garnish with additional chopped walnuts and a drizzle of brown rice syrup.

Raspberry Almond Jam Dot Cookies
Makes 3 dozen cookies

3 cups whole-wheat flour
$1/4$ teaspoon unrefined sea salt
$1/2$ cup brown rice syrup or barley malt syrup
$1/2$ cup sunflower oil
1 teaspoon almond extract
$1/2$ cup finely chopped almonds
$1/4$ to $1/2$ cup raspberry preserves

Preheat the oven to 350°F.

Mix the flour and salt well. Beat the brown rice syrup or barley malt syrup, oil, and almond extract until smooth and creamy. Combine with the flour mixture in a large bowl and blend well. Stir in the almonds. Form into 1-inch balls and place 1 to 2 inches apart on a cookie sheet. Press your thumb into each ball to flatten and make a small indentation. Bake for 10 to 15 minutes, or until golden brown. Let cool, and spoon raspberry preserves into indentations in each cookie.

Omedeto
Serves 6 to 8

Omedeto, *a traditional Japanese dessert, translates roughly to mean "congratulations rice."*

3 cups short-grain brown rice
6 cups water
$1^1/2$ cups cooked azuki beans
$1/4$ teaspoon unrefined sea salt
$1/2$ cup brown rice syrup

Toast the rice in a heavy pan until golden brown and aromatic. Add the water and cook until soft. Stir in the beans, salt, and brown rice syrup and cook over medium heat until creamy.

GLOSSARY OF TERMS AND INGREDIENTS

The following is a list of common terms and ingredients in macrobiotic cooking.

Agar-agar
Sometimes called kanten. Agar-agar is a red algae that is soaked, cooked, and pressed, then used as a thickening agent in place of gelatin. Kanten is a traditional fruit dessert made with agar-agar.

Age
Leavened tofu, deep-fried

Aka miso
Red or brown miso

Amasake
A rich, sweet beverage made from cooked brown rice fermented with koji

Arame
Thin, black seaweed used in salads, soups, and grains dishes or served as a side dish; similar in appearance to hijiki

Arrowroot
A powder from the tuber of the arrowroot plant, used as a natural thickening agent

Azuki (Aduki)
Small, compact, dark red beans originally grown in Japan

Bancha
A traditional tea made from the twigs, stems, and leaves harvested from the mature tea bush

Barley malt syrup
A natural sweetener from concentrated barley. Barley malt syrup has a rich, heavy taste, stronger than honey and sweeter than rice syrup, and is well suited for baking and heartier dishes.

Bonito flakes
A seasoning made from dried bonito fish, used in stocks or as a garnish

Brown rice miso
A type of miso made from brown rice, soybeans, and sea salt. Also known as *genmai miso*, brown rice miso is mild and sweet, and is generally used for dressings, sauces, and light broths.

Brown rice syrup
A natural sweetener made from malted brown rice, with a delicate flavor and a mild level of sweetness

Brown rice vinegar
A mild vinegar made from brown rice. Brown rice vinegar is high in amino acids (other vinegars contain only trace amounts of amino acids) and is used in cooking and to help restore the body's blood alkaline balance.

Burdock
A long, slender, dark root used in cooking and for medicinal purposes. Burdock is thought to strengthen the constitution and cleanse the blood.

Daikon
A long, cylindrical white radish used for cooking and medicinal purposes

Dashi
A traditional Japanese soup stock made from boiling kombu and water into a broth

Dulse
A tangy red seaweed used primarily in soup stocks and salads or as a garnish

Fu
Dried wheat gluten (seitan), formed into cakes or sheets

Goma
Sesame seed

Gomashio
A mixture of sesame seeds and salt in a seven-to-one ratio, used as a condiment (*shio* translates to "salt")

Hatcho miso
A type of miso made from soybeans and salt, aged for two to three years

Hijiki (Hiziki)
A dark, wiry seaweed of the brown algae family with a strong, distinctive taste; usually used in soups and grain dishes

Inari
In Oriental mythology, the god of rice

Kelp
Similar to kombu; strong-tasting seaweed that is generally used in soups and to cook grains and vegetables

Ki
Also known as *Qi* or *C'hi*. Ki is the source of movement and energy and is considered the life force in Oriental philosophy and practice. When food is consumed, it is transformed into other substances, including Ki.

Kinpira
A cooking style in which root vegetables are sautéed, then steamed and seasoned with tamari

Koji
An enzyme from grains inoculated with bacteria; used in the fermentation process to prepare such foods as miso, sake, and shoyu. *Kome koji* is fermented rice, and *mugi koji* is fermented barley.

Kombu
A broad, flat seaweed with a strong flavor and dark green color; generally used to make soup stocks and in cooking beans and grains

Kome miso
A light, milder miso made from rice and soybeans

Kukicha
A tea made from mature twigs, stems, and leaves of the tea bush

Kuzu (Kudzu)
A white starch extracted from a Japanese wild vegetable and used as a thickening agent for soups, sauces, and gravies

Maki sushi
A type of rolled sushi in which vegetables, fish, and rice are tightly rolled inside a sheet of nori seaweed, then sliced into rounds

Mirin
Similar to sake, a sweet rice wine used for cooking. To make mirin, sweet rice is combined with sake and fermented, then pressed and aged for up to two years. Mirin varies widely in quality—some kinds are made with added sugar or corn syrup—so check labels.

Miso
A fermented paste made of soybeans, salt, water, and various grains, used as a soup base and as a flavoring and condiment. Miso is available in many varieties.

Mochi
A steamed sweet rice that is pounded to a sticky dough and shaped into small blocks or flat squares. Mochi puffs up when baked and becomes soft and chewy, with a slightly sweet flavor.

Mugi miso
A type of miso made from soybeans and barley, with a mild, slightly sweet flavor

Mu tea
A traditional tea made from various herbs that are thought to have medicinal and healing properties

Nabe
A type of Japanese casserole or one-dish meal, served in a decorative casserole dish with sauces and dressings for dipping

Natto
Cooked and briefly fermented soybeans, traditionally eaten as a side dish with shoyu, ginger, daikon, mustard, or scallions, or mixed with brown rice or other grains

Natto miso
A type of miso made from soybeans, grains, ginger, and kombu, usually used as a condiment

Nigari
A coagulant agent made from the droppings of dampened sea salt; used in the preparation of tofu

Nishime
A method of cooking vegetables in which the vegetables are cut in chunks and cooked slowly over low heat for a long period of time, then seasoned with soy sauce

Nitsuke
A method of cooking vegetables in which the vegetables are cut into small pieces and cooked for a short time

Nori
A red algae seaweed, also known as purple laver. Nori is made of thin sheets of dried seaweed and is usually used for rolling sushi or making rice balls, or is toasted and crumbled as a seasoning or condiment.

Nut milks
Milks made from roasting skinned and hulled nuts, blending them with warm water until smooth, then straining

Ojiya
A porridge made with leftover rice and soup cooked together

Okara
Also called *unohana;* soybean pulp left over from the tofu-making process. Generally used in soups or for vegetable patties.

Omedeto
A ceremonial porridge prepared as dessert for special occasions and made from azuki beans and roasted brown rice

Red rice
Rice cooked with azuki beans

Rice milk
A milk substitute made from organic brown rice, with a lighter, more delicate flavor than soy milk

Sashimi
Raw fish dish

Seitan
Also called "wheat meat," made from wheat gluten cooked in shoyu, kombu, and water. Seitan has a meatlike texture and hearty flavor and is ideal for soups and stews.

Shiitake
Also known as Chinese black mushrooms. Shiitake are available fresh or dried and are used for cooking and medicinal purposes, to help neutralize animal fats and excess salt.

Shio
Salt

Shiso
Also called beefsteak leaves; a Japanese plant used for flavoring, commonly pickled with umeboshi plums

Shoyu

Made from fermented soybeans, wheat, and salt. Similar to soy sauce but generally refers to a naturally fermented soy sauce as opposed to commercial brands, which may contain sugar, corn syrup, monosodium glutamate (MSG), and other additives.

Soba

Buckwheat noodles. The word *soba,* when used as a prefix, means "buckwheat."

Soy milk

A substitute for regular milk or cream; made from cooked soybeans or the liquid residue from making tofu. Soy milk is available in many varieties, including flavored, sweetened, low salt, and calcium fortified.

Soy sauce

A traditional seasoning and condiment made from fermented soybeans, wheat, and salt. Soy sauce differs from tamari in that it contains wheat and is fermented in a different manner. Commercial soy sauce may contain chemical additives and preservatives.

Su

Vinegar

Suimono

Clear broth

Suribachi

A deep bowl with sloping sides and a ridged inner surface, used to grind seeds and make sauces and dressings; used with a wooden pestle

Surikogi

Wooden pestle used with a suribachi

Sushi

Originally fish pickled in vinegar, sushi generally refers to bite-size slices of raw or sometimes cooked fish served on small mounds of rice

Tahini

A smooth paste made from ground sesame seeds. Available either roasted or raw, tahini is primarily used as a spread on bread or to make salad dressings, desserts, and sauces.

Tamari

The liquid by-product of the making of miso, used as a seasoning; differs from shoyu and soy sauce in that it contains no wheat

Tekka
A strong, salty condiment made from hatcho miso and a variety of vegetables (including lotus root, carrot, ginger, and burdock) cooked in dark sesame oil for several hours

Tempeh
A fermented protein food made from soybeans and a special bacteria starter. Tempeh holds its flavor and texture well in casseroles, soups, and stir-fried dishes.

Tempura
A traditional style of cooking in which vegetables or meats are dipped in batter and deep-fried. Tempura is served with ginger dipping sauces and grated daikon.

Texturized Vegetable Protein (TVP)
Made from soybeans formed into flakes and granules. TVP has a meatlike texture and is best used in stews and casseroles.

Tofu
A versatile protein source made from cooked soybeans and nigari, shaped into blocks, and then used in soups, sauces, stir-fries, casseroles, dressings, and a variety of other dishes

Udon
Traditional Japanese whole-wheat noodles

Umeboshi
Small apricots or plums, pickled in salt and used as a condiment or seasoning (*ume* means plum, *boshi* means dry). Umeboshi stimulates digestion and helps maintain an alkaline blood balance. They are available whole or in paste form and are used to impart a salty, sour flavor to foods.

Wakame
A long, thin seaweed with a mild, slightly sweet taste. Wakame turns bright green after soaking and is ideal for miso broths and salads.

White miso
A mild, slightly sweet miso; also called mellow white miso

GROCERY SHOPPING LIST

THE FOLLOWING IS A LIST of the most commonly used foods in the macrobiotic kitchen—photocopy it from this book and use whenever you go shopping. And don't think that you have to purchase everything on the list—this is simply a fairly comprehensive outline of foods you may need at various times. It should change from week to week, depending on your needs.

Many grains, noodles, beans, nuts, seeds, and sea vegetables may be purchased in the bulk section of your natural-products store, as can many oils and sweeteners. All oils should be unrefined, fruits and vegetables should be organic whenever possible, and fruits may be either fresh or dried.

Most of the condiments and seasonings listed here are available at larger natural-products stores or at most Oriental food stores. If you purchase ingredients at Oriental markets, read labels carefully to check for added sugar, refined salt, monosodium glutamate (MSG), artificial preservatives, and other additives. If you can't find what you're looking for from your local vendors, check Appendix D: Mail-Order Guide and Resource List. Happy hunting!

GRAINS

barley
brown rice (long, medium, and
    short grain; basmati and
    kokuko rose)
brown rice cereal
buckwheat
corn (flour, grits, and meal)
couscous
millet
mochi
oats
quinoa
rice cream
rice cakes
rye
sweet brown rice
unleavened bread
wheat (cracked, germ, flour,
    and bulghur)
wild rice

NOODLES

saifun or cellophane
soba
somen
udon
whole-grain pastas (corn, whole-
    wheat, etc. in various shapes)

BEANS AND BEAN PRODUCTS

anasazi
azuki (aduki)
black turtle beans
chickpeas (garbanzos)
kidney beans
lentils
limas
mung beans
navy beans
pinto beans
soybeans
split peas

VEGETABLES

acorn squash
alfalfa sprouts
artichokes
asparagus
bean sprouts
beets
Belgian endive
bitter greens
bok choy
broccoli
Brussels sprouts
burdock
butternut squash
cabbage (red, green)
carrots
cauliflower
celery/celery root
Chinese cabbage
chives
collard greens
corn
cucumbers
daikon
endive
green beans
herbs, fresh (cilantro, tarragon,
    basil, rosemary, thyme, etc.)
kale
leeks
lettuce (red leaf, romaine, wild
    greens)
mushrooms, button and wild
    (morel, chanterelle, porcini,
    shiitake)
mustard greens
onions (red, yellow, and white)
parsley
parsnips
peas
pumpkin
radishes
red peppers

rutabagas
scallions
shallots
snow peas
spinach
sprouts (all varieties)
summer squash
sweet potatoes
Swiss chard
turnip greens
turnips
watercress
winter squash
zucchini

FRUITS
apples
apricots
blueberries
cantaloupe
cherries
grapes
melons (in season)
peaches
pears
plums
raisins
raspberries
strawberries

PROTEIN SOURCES
fish, white meat (carp, clams, cod, flounder, haddock, halibut, mussels, oysters, red snapper, scallops, shrimp, sole, trout)
fish, dark meat for occasional use (tuna, salmon, herring, eel, trout, shrimp, lobster, crab, squid)
rice, soy, and nut milks
rice, soy, and nut cheeses
seitan

tempeh
textured vegetable protein (TVP)
tofu (firm and silken)

NUTS AND SEEDS
almonds
black sesame seeds
chestnuts
filberts
nut/seed butters (almond, peanut, sunflower, tahini)
peanuts
pecans
pine nuts
poppyseeds
pumpkin seeds (pepitas)
sesame seeds
sunflower seeds
walnuts

SEA VEGETABLES
arame
dulse
hijiki
Irish moss
kombu
nori
wakame

OILS
almond
corn
olive
peanut
safflower
sesame (dark, light)
sunflower

CONDIMENTS AND SEASONINGS
brown rice vinegar
celery seed
garlic

ginger
gomashio
grated horseradish
mirin
miso
mustards
pepper (black, white)
pickled vegetables
roasted sea vegetables
sake
shoyu/soy sauce
tamari
tekka
umeboshi plums or paste
umeboshi vinegar
unrefined sea salt
wasabi

SWEETENERS
amasake
barley malt syrup
brown rice syrup
fruit juice
honey

BEVERAGES
bancha tea
kukicha tea
mild herbal teas
Mu tea
roasted grain teas
spring water

THE MACROBIOTIC MAKEUP

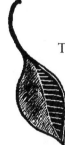

THE PROPORTION OF FOOD in the daily macrobiotic diet focuses on balance—a feat most easily achieved by consuming foods that fall near the center of the yin/yang continuum. The daily diet can be easily constructed to ensure a balance of the types, quality, and volume of foods without rigorous preparation and planning. This doesn't mean that the consumption of certain foods not in the center of the yin/yang continuum is forever forbidden—occasional, careful use of foods that fall in the macro no-nos category is permitted. In general, however, the daily diet should be based on grains, vegetables, beans, sea vegetables, unrefined vegetable oils, seeds and nuts, white-meat fish, and small amounts of seasonings and unrefined sweeteners.

GRAINS

Grains should make up 50 to 60 percent of daily meals. Include rice (long- and short-grain brown rice, rice cream, sweet brown rice, mochi, and rice crackers), millet, barley, corn, oats, wheat, rye, buckwheat, and quinoa, as well as seitan and rice milk.

VEGETABLES

Vegetables should make up about 25 to 30 percent of the daily diet. All vegetables should be cooked or lightly steamed to aid in assimilation by the body, with the exception of sprouts and lettuces. Preparation can vary from steaming, baking, and sautéing to pressure-cooking. Examples of root vegetables with a more yang influence include burdock, daikon, parsnips, rutabagas, and turnips. Leafy vegetables with a more yin influence include bok choy, Chinese cabbage, collard greens, kale, lettuces, mustard greens, spinach, and turnip greens. Vegetables that can be used regularly include asparagus, mushrooms, broccoli, Brussels sprouts, butternut squash, carrots, cauliflower, celery, cabbage, cucumber, endive, green beans, peas, leeks, onions, sprouts, summer squash, and zucchini.

Beans and Bean Products

Beans and bean products should make up about 10 percent of the daily diet. Low-fat, white-meat fish from clean sources may be eaten in moderation (two to three small portions a week). Use anasazi, azuki, black-eyed peas, garbanzos, kidney beans, lentils, limas, mung beans, navy beans, pinto beans, soybeans, and sprouts. Types of bean products to be used include tofu, tempeh, soy milk, and soy cheese.

Sea Vegetables

Sea vegetables should make up about 5 percent of the daily diet. Sea vegetables are eaten in small quantities and can be used when cooking beans and soups and as an ingredient in salads, stews, and other dishes. Use arame, dulse, hijiki, Irish moss, kombu, nori, and wakame.

Soups

Soups should make up about 3 to 5 percent of the daily diet. One to two bowls of miso soup, kombu broth, or miso/kombu-based soup should be eaten daily either at breakfast, as an appetizer or first course, or as a main meal.

Nuts and Seeds

Nuts and seeds are used sparingly and should be eaten raw as snacks or can be ground into butters or used as garnish. Include almonds, chestnuts, peanuts, pecans, pine nuts, walnuts, sesame seeds, pumpkin seeds, sunflower seeds, poppyseeds, and nut and seed butters (tahini, almond butter, sunflower butter, peanut butter).

FRUITS

Fruits can be used in the daily diet in moderation. Use locally available, organically grown fruits in season. Fruits to use include apples, apricots, berries, grapes, melons, persimmons, peaches, pears, and plums. Citrus and tropical fruits should be consumed in small amounts only in warmer weather or climates, and melons should always be eaten alone.

FISH AND SHELLFISH

Fish is eaten in small quantities two or three times a week. White-meat fish and shellfish are recommended, including flounder, haddock, halibut, snapper, trout, sole, cod, whitefish, clams, oysters, scallops, mussels, and octopus. Dark-meat, oilier fish and shellfish like tuna, swordfish, salmon, herring, eel, shrimp, lobster, crab, and squid are eaten less frequently.

CONDIMENTS AND SEASONINGS

Use condiments and seasonings sparingly. In the traditional Japanese macrobiotic diet, each meal includes a small portion of some type of pickled vegetable, such as daikon or ginger, to balance the meal and help aid the digestive process. This practice is easy to incorporate into a mostly macro diet as well.

MAIL-ORDER GUIDE AND RESOURCE LIST

MACROBIOTIC SUPPLIES/ INGREDIENTS

Gold Mine Natural Foods
3419 Hancock Street
San Diego, CA 92110
(619) 296-8536

Kushi Institute
Box 38
Becket, MA 01223
(413) 623-5741

George Ohsawa Macrobiotic Foundation
1999 Myers Street
Oroville, CA 95966
(916) 533-7702

Mountain Arc
1601 Pump Station Road
Fayetteville, AR 72701
(800) 643-8909
(501) 442-7191

Natural Life Supplies
16 Lookout Drive
Asheville, NC 28804
(704) 254-9606

ORGANIC FOODS

Community Mill and Bean
267 Route 89 South
Savannah, NY 13146
(800) 755-0554

Eagle Organic and Natural Food
P.O. Box 1451
Huntsville, AR 72740
(501) 738-2203

The Green Earth
2545 Prairie Avenue
Evanston, IL 60201
(708) 475-0205

Trading Co.
120 South East Avenue
Fayetteville, AR 72701
(501) 442-7191

Walnut Acres Organic Farms
Walnut Acres Road
Penns Creek, PA 17862
(800) 433-3998

BIBLIOGRAPHY

Aihara, Cornelia, and Herman Aihara. *Natural Healing from Head to Toe.* Garden City Park, NY: Avery Publishing, 1994.

Aihara, Herman. *Basic Macrobiotics.* Tokyo, Japan: Japan Publications, 1985.

Belleme, John, and Jan Belleme. *Cooking With Japanese Foods.* Garden City Park, NY: Avery Publishing, 1993.

Dufty, William. *Sugar Blues.* New York: Warner Books, 1975.

Esko, Edward, and Wendy Esko. *Macrobiotic Cooking for Everyone.* Tokyo, Japan: Japan Publications, 1980.

Esko, Wendy. *Introducing Macrobiotic Cooking.* Tokyo, Japan: Japan Publications, 1978.

Heidenry, Carolyn. *An Introduction to Macrobiotics.* Garden City Park, NY: Avery Publishing, 1987.

———. *Making the Transition to a Macrobiotic Diet.* Garden City Park, NY: Avery Publishing, 1987.

Kushi, Aveline. *How to Cook With Miso.* Tokyo, Japan: Japan Publications, 1979.

Kushi, Aveline, and Alex Jack. *Aveline Kushi's Complete Guide to Macrobiotic Cooking for Health, Harmony, and Peace.* New York: Warner Books, 1985.

Kushi, Aveline, and Michio Kushi. *Macrobiotic Diet.* Tokyo and New York: Japan Publications, 1993.

Kushi, Aveline, and Wendy Esko. *Aveline Kushi's Introducing Macrobiotic Cooking.* Garden City Park, NY: Avery Publishing, 1985.

———. *Macrobiotic Family Favorites*. Tokyo, Japan: Japan Publications, 1987.

Kushi, Michio. *The Macrobiotic Way*. Garden City Park, NY: Avery Publishing, 1993.

Michell, Keith. *Practically Macrobiotic*. Rochester, VT: Healing Arts Press, 1988.

Nishimoto, Miyoko. *The Now and Zen Epicure*. Summertown, TN: Book Publishing Company, 1991.

Ohsawa, George. *Macrobiotic Guide Book for Living*. Los Angeles: Ohsawa Foundation, 1966.

Sams, Craig. *The Macrobiotic Brown Rice Cookbook*. Rochester, VT: Healing Arts Press, 1993.

Turner, Kristina. *The Self-Healing Cookbook*. Vashon Island, WA: Earthtones Press, 1989.

Weber, Marcea, and Daniel Weber. *Macrobiotics and Beyond*. Dorset, England: Prism Press, 1988.

INDEX